The

Intensive Care Nurse

The Complete Guide

ALEXANDRE CAREWELL

Table of Contents

« *Faced with the fragility of life, the intensive care nurse is the silent guardian of hope, working tirelessly to transform every breath into a possible future.* »

Chapter 1:
INTRODUCTION TO INTENSIVE CARE

History and development of resuscitation

Resuscitation, this intense medical practice aimed at supporting or restoring vital functions, has its roots in human history, long before the advanced technology we know today. Each stage in its development reveals a facet of our ceaseless quest to defy death and give life a second chance.

Let's go back to the 18th century, when Europe was fascinated by the phenomenon of 'resuscitating' drowning victims. It was at this time that societies, such as the Royal Humane Society in England, were formed with the main aim of promoting techniques for reviving drowning victims. They encouraged the use of methods, now considered primitive, such as warming the body, draining water from the lungs or even blowing tobacco smoke into the lungs!

The 19th century saw the advent of the first forms of intubation, a crucial advance in the management of obstructed airways. But it was in the 20th century that resuscitation really took off. After the horrors of the First and Second World Wars, the need to treat large numbers of wounded led to significant advances in emergency medicine and surgery, laying the foundations for modern resuscitation.

The 1950s marked a decisive stage with the advent of mechanical ventilation, mainly in response to the polio epidemic. These ventilators, although archaic by today's standards, saved many lives and paved the way for the specialist intensive care units we know today.

The advent of technology and research over the last few decades has revolutionised resuscitation. Advanced cardiac monitors, defibrillators, dialysis and advances in pharmacology have made it possible to save patients who, just a few years ago, would have had no chance of survival. Resuscitation has become an interdisciplinary collaboration, combining the skills of doctors, nurses, physiotherapists and many other professionals, each making their own contribution to providing the best possible care.

Today, intensive care units represent the pinnacle of clinical medicine, skilfully blending cutting-edge technology, clinical skills and compassion. But technology and science aside, resuscitation reminds us of a universal constant: our resolute determination to preserve life, to understand the delicate balance between life and death, and to always seek ways to improve this delicate art.

This historical legacy reminds us of the importance of resuscitation in our society and lays the foundations for understanding its crucial role and impact on medical care today and in the future.

The importance of Intensive Care

Intensive Care, more than just a hospital ward, embodies the intersection of advanced medical technology, clinical expertise, and deep humanity in the world of healthcare. At the heart of the hospital, the Intensive Care Unit (ICU) is often the last resort for patients whose lives are in danger. Its place and importance are undeniable, both from a medical and a societal point of view.

From a purely clinical point of view, the ICU specialises in the care of the most critical patients, those whose one or more organs are not functioning properly or are failing. This could be the heart, lungs, kidneys or even the brain. Intensive care combines constant monitoring with complex medical interventions to stabilise, treat and hopefully reverse these organ failures. Patients who would once have been lost to insurmountable medical challenges may now have a chance of recovery, thanks to the skills and technologies deployed in resuscitation.

As well as technology and clinical expertise, intensive care is also essential on a human level. The ICU is often the scene of intense emotions, where hope and despair, joy and grief come together. It is a reminder of the fragility of life and the need for holistic care, taking into account not only the patient, but also his or her family and loved ones. The importance of clear communication, emotional support and a deep respect for the wishes and needs of the patient and their family is paramount.

In societal terms, intensive care is also a reflection of our collective values. How do we allocate scarce medical resources? How do we balance the objective of prolonging life with the quality of that life? How do we navigate the murky waters of medical ethics, taking into account patients' wishes, rights and dignity? These crucial questions arise daily in intensive care and shape our collective approach to medicine and morality.

Finally, intensive care is also of strategic importance in terms of public health. Whether during epidemics, natural disasters or other crises, the ICU plays a pivotal role in the response of our healthcare system. Recent events, such as the COVID-19 pandemic, have highlighted the vital importance of intensive care in managing health crises.

The importance of Intensive Care cannot be underestimated. It is both a feat of modern medicine and a testament to our commitment to human life, dignity and health. Every moment spent in the ICU is a reminder of the importance of compassion, innovation and excellence in the pursuit of healing.

Definition and specific features the Intensive Care Unit

The Intensive Care Unit (ICU) is much more than just a hospital ward: it is the beating heart of emergency medicine, a front line dedicated to combating the most serious vital failures and life-threatening conditions. The unit combines technology, clinical expertise and human care to provide comprehensive care for patients in critical condition.

Definition of ICU :
The ICU is a specialised hospital facility designed to monitor, diagnose and treat patients with acute failure of one or more organ systems. These patients require continuous monitoring, intensive medical interventions and often technological assistance to support their vital functions.

Special features of the ICU :
- **State-of-the-art equipment:** The ICU is equipped with advanced medical devices, including heart monitors, respirators and dialysis machines, among others. This equipment not only allows us to monitor patients' vital signs in real time, but also to provide life-saving assistance when their organs can no longer function properly.
- **Specialist staff:** The ICU is staffed by a team of highly qualified professionals, including intensive care physicians, intensive care nurses, physiotherapists, nutritionists and other specialists, all trained to meet the specific needs of critically ill patients.
- **Comprehensive care:** Beyond simple monitoring, the ICU offers a holistic approach to care, including

surgical interventions, advanced pharmacological treatments, appropriate nutritional support and psychological care for patients and their families.

- **Controlled environment:** The ICU environment is carefully regulated in terms of cleanliness, noise levels and lighting, to minimise stress for patients and optimise healing conditions.
- **Ethics and communication: Due to the** seriousness of the cases treated in the ICU, complex ethical issues often arise. The ICU is therefore characterised by transparent and respectful communication with patients and their families, and particular attention is paid to advance directives, informed consent and end-of-life decisions.
- **Research and innovation:** ICUs are often at the forefront of medical research, exploring new treatment methods, drugs and technologies to improve survival rates and quality of care for critically ill patients.

The Intensive Care Unit is therefore a unique space, combining medical expertise and humanity, to offer a second chance to those who need it most. It is both a symbol of the progress of modern medicine and a constant reminder of the fragile interconnection between life, death and science.

Chapter 2:
THE FUNDAMENTALS
OF THE INTENSIVE CARE NURSE

Anatomy and physiology : essential reminders

To fully understand the importance and complexity of the Intensive Care Unit, it is crucial to have a sound knowledge of the fundamentals of anatomy and physiology. These disciplines provide an in-depth understanding of the structure and function of our bodies, two inextricably linked elements, and serve as the basis for everything that is undertaken in the ICU.

1. Respiratory system :
   * **Anatomy:** Comprising the upper (nose, mouth, pharynx, larynx) and lower (trachea, bronchi, lungs) airways. The pulmonary alveoli are the small pockets of air where gas exchange takes place.
   * **Physiology:** Ensures oxygenation of the blood by inhaling oxygen and exhaling carbon dioxide. The respiratory mechanism is regulated by the respiratory centre located in the brain.

2. Cardiovascular system :
   * **Anatomy:** The heart is the main organ, acting like a pump to propel blood through a complex network of vessels (arteries, veins and capillaries).
   * **Physiology:** Supplies every cell in the body with oxygen and essential nutrients, while eliminating waste products such as carbon dioxide and urea.

3. Renal system :
- **Anatomy:** Mainly made up of the kidneys, ureters, bladder and urethra.
- **Physiology:** Filters and eliminates waste products from the blood, regulates water and electrolyte balance, and produces urine.

4. Nervous system :
- **Anatomy:** Divided into the central nervous system (brain and spinal cord) and the peripheral nervous system (nerves and ganglia).
- **Physiology:** Regulates and coordinates the body's activities, detects and interprets external and internal stimuli, and generates appropriate responses.

5. Digestive system :
- **Anatomy:** Includes the mouth, oesophagus, stomach, small intestine, large intestine, liver, gallbladder and pancreas.
- **Physiology:** Transformation of food into absorbable nutrients to provide energy and support cell growth.

6. Endocrine system :
- **Anatomy: A** group of glands (thyroid, parathyroid, adrenal glands, pancreas, pituitary gland, etc.) which produce hormones.
- **Physiology:** Regulation of various bodily functions, such as metabolism, growth, development and response to stress, through the secretion of hormones.

7. Immune system :
- **Anatomy:** Includes the thymus, bone marrow, lymph nodes, spleen and network of lymphatic vessels.
- **Physiology:** Protects the body against infection and disease by recognising and eliminating pathogens.

By immersing ourselves in these systems and understanding their interrelationships, we gain a deep appreciation of the complexity of the human body. In the Intensive Care Unit, this knowledge is essential. Failures in any one of these systems can have cascading repercussions, requiring rapid and specialised intervention to stabilise the patient and promote recovery.

Common diseases in intensive care

Resuscitation, being at the forefront of the management of the most serious medical cases, treats a variety of pathologies. Whether they are acute conditions resulting from a sudden event or complications of a chronic illness, the Intensive Care Unit is equipped to manage these situations. Here is an overview of the pathologies frequently encountered in intensive care:

1. Acute respiratory failure :
   - **Causes:** Pneumonia, pulmonary oedema, COPD exacerbation, severe asthma, pulmonary embolism, ARDS (acute respiratory distress syndrome).

2. Shock and haemodynamic failure :
   - **Causes:** septic shock (due to a serious infection), cardiogenic shock (heart problems), haemorrhagic shock (heavy blood loss), anaphylactic shock (severe allergic reaction).

3. Severe neurological disorders :
   - **Causes:** Stroke, head trauma, meningitis, encephalitis, uncontrolled epilepsy.

4. Acute renal failure :**Causes:** Glomerulonephritis, nephrotoxicity (due to certain drugs or toxins), renal ischaemia, complications of systemic pathologies.

5. Sepsis and severe infections :
   - **Origin:** Bacterial, viral, fungal or parasitic infections that spread through the bloodstream. Common sources include pneumonia, meningitis, urinary tract infections or post-operative infections.

6. Multiple trauma :
   - **Causes:** Road accidents, falls from height, blunt trauma, gunshot or stab wounds.

7. Post-operative complications :
   - **Causes:** Complications following heart surgery, transplantation, major surgery of the thorax or abdomen, or after surgery with a risk of complications.

8. Multiple organ failure :
   - **Origin:** Progression of one of the above conditions or as a result of sepsis, severe inflammation or ischaemia affecting several organs.

9. Serious metabolic and endocrine disorders :
   - **Causes:** diabetic ketoacidosis, hyperosmolar coma, thyrotoxic crisis (thyroid storm), addisonian crisis.

10. Acute poisoning :
   - **Causes:** Drug overdoses, ingestion of toxic substances, carbon monoxide poisoning.

Every intensive care patient presents a unique set of challenges based on their pathology, medical history and individual needs. Management often requires an interdisciplinary approach, combining medicine, surgery, pharmacology, physiotherapy and other specialities to provide the best possible care.

Vital parameters : monitoring and interpretation

Monitoring vital parameters is fundamental in intensive care. These measurements provide an instant overview of the patient's stability and physiological well-being. Regular monitoring and correct interpretation enable complications to be anticipated, interventions to be guided and the patient's progress to be monitored.

1. Heart rate (HR) :
   - **Monitoring:** Using a heart monitor, pulse oximeter or manually at a pulse point.
   - **Interpretation:** A high heart rate (tachycardia) may indicate fever, dehydration, haemorrhage or a response to stress. Low heart rate (bradycardia) may be normal in some individuals, or indicate a heart problem, drug overdose or increased intracranial pressure.

2. Blood pressure (BP) :
   - **Monitoring:** With an automatic blood pressure monitor or arterial catheter for continuous invasive measurement.
   - **Interpretation:** High blood pressure may indicate pain, a response to stress, or cardiac pathology. Low blood pressure may indicate haemorrhage,
   - heart failure or septicaemia.

3. Respiratory rate (RR) :
   - **Monitoring:** Direct observation of the rise and fall of the ribcage or via a sensor on the patient monitor.

- **Interpretation:** A high FR (tachypnoea) may be due to respiratory distress, acidosis or fever. A low FR (bradypnoea) could indicate drug overdose, respiratory fatigue or neurological impairment.

4. Temperature :
   - **Monitoring:** Ear, mouth, rectal or skin thermometer.
   - **Interpretation:** Fever often suggests infection, inflammation or a response to certain drugs. A low temperature (hypothermia) may result from exposure to cold, sepsis or adrenal insufficiency.

5. Oxygen saturation (SpO2) :
   - **Monitoring:** Via a pulse oximeter usually placed on the finger, ear or foot.
   - **Interpretation:** A low SpO2 indicates hypoxaemia, which may be due to respiratory failure, pulmonary embolism or a cardiac shunt.

6. Pain scale :
   - **Monitoring:** Using standardised scales or simply by interviewing the patient.
   - **Interpretation:** Pain can influence other vital parameters, and its management is essential for comfort and recovery.

7. State of consciousness :
   - **Monitoring:** Via Glasgow Scale or AVPU assessment (Alert, Voice Response, Pain Response, Non-Reactive).
   - **Interpretation:** An alteration may indicate brain damage, intoxication, hypoxia or hypoglycaemia, among other things.

Regular and accurate monitoring of these parameters is essential. A rapid or unexpected change in one of these vital signs may be the first indication of an imminent complication, requiring immediate intervention. In intensive care, where every second counts, mastery of the monitoring and interpretation of vital parameters is an invaluable skill.

Chapter 3:
TECHNIQUES
AND SPECIFIC INTERVENTIONS

Route of administration
and catheter management

In the intensive care unit, the rapid and efficient administration of drugs and other solutions can be vital to a patient's survival. This requires a thorough knowledge of the different routes of administration and an impeccable command of catheter management.

1. Route of administration :
   - **Oral route:** Although often preferred for its simplicity, this route may not be possible due to the patient's condition (coma, intubation) or the nature of the drug.
   - **Intravenous (IV):** This provides direct access to the bloodstream, allowing rapid action of the drugs.
   - **Intraosseous (IO):** Used when rapid intravenous access is necessary but difficult to obtain. It involves inserting a needle into the bone marrow.
   - **Subcutaneous route:** Mainly for administering insulin or anticoagulants.
   - **Intramuscular route:** Allows the drug to be absorbed more slowly than with IV administration.
   - **Transdermal:** Using patches that release the drug into the bloodstream through the skin.
   - **Inhaled route:** For medicines designed to act directly on the respiratory tract, such as bronchodilators.

2. Catheter management :
- Peripheral venous catheter :
    - **Insertion:** Choice of site depending on the patient's anatomy and the expected duration of the infusion.
    - **Care:** Regular dressing changes, monitoring for signs of infection or phlebitis, maintaining strict asepsis.
- Central venous catheter (CVC) :
    - **Insertion:** Under ultrasound guidance to reduce complications. Common sites: internal jugular vein, subclavian vein and femoral vein.
    - **Care:** Sterile dressing, monitoring for signs of infection, regular checking of position by X-ray.
- Arterial catheter :
    - **Insertion:** Often into the radial or femoral artery, to monitor blood pressure or take blood samples.
    - **Care:** Monitoring the distal perfusion, maintaining sterility, checking the pressure curve.
- Swan-Ganz catheter or thermodilution catheter :
    - **Insertion:** Measures cardiac pressures and mixed oxygen saturation.
    - **Care:** Regular calibration, monitoring of haemodynamic parameters, prevention of infections.
- Dialysis catheter :
    - **Insertion:** For haemodialysis or continuous glomerular filtration.
    - **Care:** Monitoring for signs of infection, assessing catheter function, maintaining asepsis.

Catheter management in intensive care requires extensive training and regular updating of skills to prevent complications. Proper handling, rigorous monitoring and understanding of each type of catheter are essential to ensure patient safety and well-being.

Respiratory assistance : non-invasive ventilation intubation

In resuscitation, when a patient's lungs cannot provide sufficient oxygen to the body or properly remove carbon dioxide, respiratory support can be vital. The management of patients requiring respiratory support has progressed considerably over the decades, from less invasive methods to more complex interventions such as intubation.

1. Non-invasive ventilation (NIV) :
   - **Purpose and indications :** NIV supports respiratory function without having to insert a tube into the trachea. It is often used for COPD exacerbations, cardiogenic pulmonary oedema and certain types of pneumonia.
   - CPAP (Continuous Positive Airway Pressure) :
     - Continuous positive airway pressure (CPAP) keeps the airways open and is commonly used to treat sleep apnea and pulmonary oedema.
   - BiPAP (Bilevel Positive Airway Pressure) :
     - Unlike CPAP, BiPAP offers different inhalation and exhalation pressures, providing better support for those who find it difficult to exhale against positive pressure.

2. Indications for intubation :
Reasons why a patient may require intubation include acute respiratory distress, airway protection (e.g. during surgery), inability to remove CO_2 or hypoventilation.

3. Intubation procedure :
- **Preparation:** Ensure venous access, administer appropriate sedation and analgesics, and sometimes paralysing agents. Position the patient in the sniffing position.
- **Technique:** Using a laryngoscope, the doctor visualises the vocal cords and inserts the endotracheal tube. Confirmation of the position is vital, and is usually performed using capnography and auscultation.
- **Potential complications:** These include an incorrectly positioned tube, damage to the vocal cords, oesophageal intubation or pneumothorax.

4. Mechanical ventilation :
After intubation, the patient is often connected to a mechanical ventilator, which can be set to different modes depending on the patient's needs, such as assisted/controlled ventilation (ACV) or ventilation with a predefined volume or pressure.

5. Weaning and extubation :
Weaning is the process of gradually reducing the patient's dependence on mechanical ventilation. It must be carefully planned and executed. Extubation, or removal of the tube, occurs when the patient is able to breathe effectively on his own.

The management of respiratory distress is complex and requires coordination between doctors, nurses, respiratory physiotherapists and other members of the care team. A thorough understanding of respiratory assessment, the indications for each mode of assistance and possible complications is essential to ensure optimal management in intensive care.

Complication management and emergency situations

In the intensive care unit, every moment can turn into an emergency situation. Nurses and all medical staff must therefore be prepared to intervene quickly and effectively. Success in managing complications depends on the ability to recognise early warning signs, have a thorough understanding of the potential aetiology and implement an appropriate intervention plan.

1. Cardiac arrest :
   - **Recognition:** Absence of pulse, consciousness and breathing.
   - **Intervention:** Immediate initiation of cardiopulmonary resuscitation (CPR), defibrillation if indicated, administration of medication according to the ACLS (Advanced Cardiac Life Support) protocol.

2. Acute respiratory distress :
   - **Possible causes:** pulmonary oedema, pneumothorax, pulmonary embolism, aspiration.
   - **Intervention:** oxygenation, ventilation adjustments, possibly intubation or thoracic paracentesis.

3. Septic shock :
   - **Recognition:** Hypotension, tachycardia, altered consciousness, oliguria.
   - **Intervention:** Rapid administration of fluids, antibiotics, haemodynamic monitoring, possibly vasopressors.

4. Internal or external bleeding :
   - **Recognition:** Hypotension, tachycardia, pallor, anxiety, visible bleeding.

- **Intervention:** Stop bleeding, fluid resuscitation, blood transfusion if necessary.

5. Neurological complications :
   - **Examples:** stroke, intracranial haemorrhage, cerebral hernia.
   - **Intervention:** Stabilisation, CT scan, monitoring of intracranial pressure, surgery if necessary.

6. Metabolic complications :
   - **Examples:** Hyperkalaemia, hypoglycaemia, metabolic acidosis.
   - **Intervention:** Correction of the anomaly using medication, dialysis or other corrective measures.

7. Equipment-related complications :
   - **Examples:** Displacement of the endotracheal tube, obstruction of the catheter, ventilator malfunction.
   - **Intervention:** Rapid reassessment of equipment, correction or replacement, continuous monitoring.

8. Infectious complications :
   - **Recognition:** Fever, chills, changes in laboratory tests, symptoms specific to the organ affected.
   - **Intervention:** Cultures, targeted antibiotics, isolation measures.

Every complication or emergency requires a systematic approach, guided by a thorough clinical assessment and, often, rapid diagnostic tests. The key is rapid but considered action, effective communication with the team and constant updating of skills and knowledge through ongoing training. In an environment as dynamic as the intensive care unit, preparation is essential.

Chapter 4:
THE ART OF COMMUNICATION IN INTENSIVE CARE

Communication with the intubated patient or under sedation

The ability to communicate is a fundamental human need. However, in intensive care, patients who are intubated or sedated often find themselves in a situation where speech is temporarily withdrawn. For nurses, ensuring effective communication with these patients is not only essential for optimal clinical management, but also for the patient's emotional and psychological well-being.

1. The importance of communication :
   - **Reducing anxiety:** The inability to speak or move freely can cause intense stress. Reassuring the patient by communicating is essential.
   - **Gathering information:** Even without speech, a patient can provide vital information about their pain, discomfort or other needs.

2. Non-verbal methods :
   - **Lip-reading:** If the patient is able to move their lips without making a sound, lip-reading may be an option.
   - **Sign language:** Simple gestures, such as a thumbs-up for "yes" or a shake of the head for "no", can be agreed.
   - **Communication board:** A board with commonly used words, letters or symbols for the patient to point to.

- **Writing:** If the patient has sufficient strength and coordination, they can write down their needs or questions.

3. Use of technology :
   - **Tablets or smartphones:** Specific applications can make communication easier, particularly text-to-speech applications.
   - **Lights or bells:** A simple system for alerting staff can be put in place.

4. Interpreting non-verbal signals :
   - **Facial expressions:** A grimace may indicate pain, a frown confusion.
   - **Gestures:** Gestures such as grabbing your chest can signal chest pain.
   - **Body language:** Restlessness, fidgeting or other movements may indicate discomfort or an unmet need.

5. Ensuring a human presence :
   - **Touch:** A hand held, a caress on the forehead or a simple touch can offer comfort and reassurance.
   - **Talking:** Even if the patient can't talk back, talking regularly, explaining what's happening, playing favourite music or playing the voice of a loved one can be comforting.

6. Preparing for communication :
   - **Training for carers:** Nurses should receive specific training in communicating with non-verbal patients.
   - **Family involvement:** Family members can often interpret subtle signals that medical staff may miss.

Communication with an intubated or sedated patient is challenging, but remains an essential aspect of resuscitation management. Recognising the patient's need to express themselves and understand, and implementing strategies to facilitate this communication, can greatly improve their experience in intensive care.

Working with the medical team: doctors, Caregivers, and other professionals

The intensive care unit is a complex environment where patients' lives depend on rapid, precise and coordinated interventions. For nurses, working closely with a multidisciplinary team is fundamental. This collaboration guarantees not only patient safety, but also optimal overall care.

1. Understanding roles :
   - **Doctors:** They make the diagnosis, define the treatment plan and are often the focal point for coordinating care.
   - **Caregivers :** They assist with basic care, such as hygiene, mobilisation and nutrition.
   - **Other professionals:** physiotherapists, nutritionists, pharmacists, psychologists, etc., bring their specific expertise to the table to provide comprehensive care.

2. Effective communication :
   - **Targeted communications:** providing accurate and relevant information during communications to ensure continuity of care.
   - **Multidisciplinary meetings:** These regular meetings are used to discuss complex cases and ensure that all professionals are aligned.

3. Defending the patient's needs :
- **Advocacy:** The nurse is often the patient's main advocate, ensuring that their needs and preferences are taken into account.
- **Anticipation:** Anticipating the patient's needs and communicating with the team to ensure that the necessary resources are in place.

4. Conflict management :
- **Recognition:** Quickly identify a disagreement or tension and resolve it.
- **Negotiation:** finding common solutions that respect each person's expertise while prioritising the patient's well-being.

5. Ongoing training and education :
- **Interprofessional training:** Learning together promotes a better understanding of each other's roles.
- **Workshops and simulations:** Recreate complex scenarios to practise collaboration in real-life situations.

6. Mutual support :
- **Team well-being:** Acknowledge that each member of the team may experience stress or fatigue. Offer support and ask for help if necessary.
- **Feedback:** Constructive feedback enables the team to continually improve.

7. Shared documentation :
- **Electronic medical records:** Ensuring that information is up-to-date, accessible and understandable to all team members.
- **Protocols and guidelines:** Having clear, shared guidelines ensures that all team members are on the same wavelength.

Collaboration in the intensive care unit is not just desirable; it is vital. Nurses, at the heart of this dynamic, must not only excel in their own skills, but also know how to interact, communicate and collaborate with a multitude of professionals. It is by making the most of each expertise that patient care will be most effective.

Navigating difficult situations: bereaved families, delicate announcements

One of the most delicate aspects of working in an intensive care unit is managing moments of intense emotion, whether due to shocking news, a bleak prognosis or the death of a patient. For nurses, this requires a combination of compassion, tact and skill.

1. Understanding the stages of bereavement :
   - **Denial:** The first reaction is often disbelief. It is essential to give the family time to process the information.
   - **Anger:** Misunderstanding can lead to anger. The nurse must remain calm and supportive, without taking this anger personally.
   - **Merchanting, depression, acceptance:** Recognising these stages can help nurses offer appropriate support.

2. Announce the news :
   - **Preparation:** Prepare yourself mentally, choose a quiet, private place and make sure the time is right.
   - **Clarity and honesty:** Use simple language, avoid medical jargon, and be honest about the prognosis.
   - **Empathy: Showing** empathy, listening rather than talking and allowing the family to express their feelings.

3. Managing emotional reactions :
   - **Active listening:** Lending an attentive ear, recognising the family's emotions and offering support.
   - **Reassurance without false hope: It**'s crucial to be realistic while offering reassurance.

4. Involving the care team :
   - **Specialist intervention:** If available, call in a psychosocial support team or social worker to help the family.
   - **Debriefing:** Talk to the medical team to make sure everyone is aware of the situation and to receive support.

5. Respecting rituals and beliefs :
   - **Knowledge:** Find out about the family's cultural or religious beliefs and rituals and respect them as far as possible.
   - **Flexibility:** Adapting care and support to the needs of the family.

6. Taking care of yourself :
   - **Acknowledging your emotions: It's** normal for nurses to feel emotions. It is essential to accept them and find ways of managing them.
   - **Decompression:** Find time to relax, talk to colleagues or a professional, and practise relaxation techniques.

7. Bereavement support :
   - **Memorial:** If appropriate, help the family organise a memorial or ceremony at the hospital.
   - **Follow-up:** In some establishments, follow-up with the family may be offered to provide additional support.

Difficult situations in the intensive care unit are inevitable, but with an empathetic, informed and caring approach, nurses can make a significant difference to patients and their families.

Chapter 5:
EMOTIONAL MANAGEMENT
AND WELL-BEING

Understanding burn-out,
compassion fatigue
and post-traumatic stress

The intensive care unit, with its frenetic pace and often critical situations, is a melting pot of intense emotions. For carers, working there means not only facing medical challenges, but also emotional and psychological ones. Three phenomena are particularly notable: burn-out, compassion fatigue and post-traumatic stress.

Burn-out is often mentioned in the medical field. It's a feeling of professional exhaustion, in which carers experience profound fatigue, growing demotivation and a sense of inefficiency. At the heart of this phenomenon is a loss of meaning. The day-to-day tasks seem insurmountable, the distance grows between the professional and his or her patients, and the passion that used to drive the work fades.

Related to, but distinct from, burn-out, **compassion fatigue** occurs when carers become emotionally exhausted as a result of being exposed to the suffering of others. It's as if the capacity for empathy, the fine quality that makes many carers excellent professionals, becomes a double-edged sword. By dint of feeling, sympathising and accompanying, a heaviness sets in. Patients' stories are no longer isolated anecdotes, but a cumulative weight that weighs heavily on the heart.

And then there's **post-traumatic stress**. In intensive care, it's not uncommon to witness traumatic situations, unexpected deaths and decisions with far-reaching consequences. These events, even if you are trained to deal with them, can leave their mark. Like a distant echo, they come back in the form of flashbacks, insomnia or dull anxiety.

But understanding these phenomena is already a step towards managing them. It means recognising that vulnerability is not a weakness, but a human reality. In their quest to help, Caregivers must not forget to help themselves. Strategies can be put in place, whether it's finding a balance between professional and personal life, talking to colleagues or seeking professional support.

The beauty of the caring profession lies in this gift of self, this ability to be there for others. But to continue to give, you also need to know how to fill yourself up, recharge your batteries and, sometimes, accept that the pain you feel is the reflection of a deeply committed humanity.

Resilience techniques and self-care

Faced with the harrowing realities of the intensive care unit, it is imperative for carers to develop resilience mechanisms and practise self-care. These methods are not signs of weakness, but rather tools for preserving and strengthening mental, emotional and physical health.

1. Understanding resilience :
Resilience is not the absence of emotion in the face of adversity, but the ability to bounce back from difficult situations. It involves recognising your emotions, processing them and finding ways to keep moving forward.

2. Cultivating mindfulness :
Practising meditation or mindfulness enables you to stay anchored in the present moment. It helps to distance oneself from negative emotions, manage stress better and increase tolerance to emotional pain.

3. Setting limits :
Learning to say "no" or to ask for help is essential. Knowing how to recognise your limits and giving yourself permission to take a break is crucial in preventing burn-out.

4. Physical care :
Exercise, a balanced diet and sufficient sleep are the foundations of good health. They help combat stress, improve mood and strengthen the immune system.

5. Seeking support :
Talking about your experiences and emotions to colleagues, friends or therapists can be a great help. Support groups, whether formal or informal, offer a safe space to share and feel understood.

6. Regenerative activities :
Everyone needs to find something that resources them. This could be reading, art, music, spending time with loved ones, nature, etc. These activities allow you to disconnect, regenerate and regain energy.

7. Journaling :
Writing regularly allows you to express your thoughts and emotions, reflect on the situations you've experienced and find solutions or new perspectives.

8. Further training :
Training in stress management, communication or relaxation techniques can be very beneficial. They offer practical tools for dealing with the challenges of the job.

9. Celebrating success:
Even small victories are worth celebrating. They remind us of the ultimate goal of this profession: to help and heal.

10. Gratitude :
Practising gratitude, even in the darkest moments, has been shown to have positive effects on mental health. This can be done mentally, in writing or out loud.
The key is to recognise that taking care of yourself is not a luxury, but a necessity. In a profession as demanding as intensive care, where so much is given of oneself, it's imperative to remember that you can't draw from a dry well. Resilience and self-care are the means by which we ensure that this well is always replenished.

Peer support
and the importance of debriefing

In the demanding world of intensive care, links between professionals are more essential than ever. Beyond protocols and techniques, the human element remains at the heart of the profession. In this environment, where decisions have far-reaching consequences and emotions run high, peer support and debriefing are crucial tools.

1. The power of peer support :
Working in an intensive care unit is intrinsically stressful. Nurses, doctors and other professionals regularly witness stressful situations. In this context, being able to turn to a colleague who understands the complexity of these moments is invaluable.
- **Mutual understanding:** Who else can better understand the pressure of a difficult intubation, the sadness of losing a patient or the frustration of a complicated situation than a colleague who has been through the same thing?

- **Sharing strategies:** Talking with peers not only allows you to share emotions, but also coping strategies, tips and advice.

2. The importance of debriefing :
Debriefing, often carried out after significant or traumatic events, allows the team to come together to discuss the situation.
- **Expressing and managing emotions:** After a critical event, it's crucial to be able to verbalise your feelings, be they fear, guilt, anger or anything else.
- **Analysing the situation:** Debriefing is not just emotional. It's also an opportunity to revisit the decisions made, evaluate the actions taken and consider future improvements.
- **Strengthening team cohesion:** Getting together, sharing a moment of vulnerability, strengthens the bonds between team members. This creates a working environment based on trust and mutual respect.

3. Setting up regular support :
You shouldn't wait for a crisis to occur before supporting or debriefing each other. The best thing is to set up regular mechanisms, such as :
- **Regular team meetings:** These can be used to discuss cases, share concerns or celebrate successes.
- **Debriefing training:** All team members should be trained in this practice, so that they can benefit fully from it.
- **Creating an open environment:** Encouraging a culture where the expression of emotions is accepted and where discussion is encouraged.

In a field as demanding as intensive care, solidarity and mutual support are not just assets: they are vital. They help to keep things in balance, guarantee optimum quality of care and ensure the well-being of those on the front line, day after day.

Chapter 6:
REAL CASE STUDIES :
LEARNING FROM EXPERIENCE

Acute respiratory failure

In intensive care, the failure of an organ or system can rapidly lead to a chain of complications. Acute respiratory failure, in particular, is one of the most common and critical medical emergencies requiring rapid and effective intervention.

1. Definition :
Acute respiratory failure is defined as the inability of the lungs to maintain adequate levels of oxygenation and/or correct elimination of carbon dioxide. It may be hypoxaemic (lack of oxygen) or hypercapnic (excess carbon dioxide).

2. Common causes :
Acute respiratory failure can occur for a variety of reasons, including:
   * Pneumonia
   * Acute pulmonary oedema
   * Severe asthma
   * Pulmonary embolism
   * ARDS (acute respiratory distress syndrome)
   * Thoracic trauma
   * Inhalation of fumes or chemicals

3. Clinical signs :
Symptoms can vary depending on the cause and severity, but generally include:
   * Dyspnoea (difficulty breathing)

- Cyanosis (bluish tinge to the skin, especially around the lips and nails)
- Tachypnoea (rapid breathing)
- Use of accessory muscles for breathing
- Impaired consciousness
- Sweats

4. Intensive care unit management :

Speed and efficiency are essential in stabilising a patient with acute respiratory failure.

- **Initial assessment:** As with any medical emergency, the first step is an ABCD (Airway, Breathing, Circulation, Disability) assessment to ensure the airway is clear, assess breathing, check circulation and assess level of consciousness.
- **Oxygen therapy:** The administration of oxygen is often necessary to increase oxygen intake. This can be done via a mask, nasal cannula or, in severe cases, mechanical ventilation.
- **Specific treatment:** Management will depend on the underlying cause of the failure. This may include medication, such as bronchodilators for asthma, antibiotics for pneumonia, or diuretics for pulmonary oedema.
- **Continuous monitoring:** In intensive care, monitoring is essential. This includes regular measurement of blood gases, monitoring of oxygen saturation, assessment of work of breathing and listening to the lungs.

Acute respiratory failure is a medical emergency requiring expertise, rapid decision-making and close collaboration between all healthcare professionals. In the intensive care unit, the aim is not only to stabilise the patient, but also to treat the underlying cause in order to avoid further complications.

Management of septic shock

Septic shock is one of the most severe medical emergencies and is often encountered in intensive care. It is a complication of infection that can lead to multiple organ failure and death if not treated quickly and appropriately. Understanding and prompt management of this syndrome is essential to improve survival rates.

1. Understanding septic shock :
Septic shock is triggered by an infection that leads to a systemic inflammatory response throughout the body. This response can lead to reduced cardiac output and poor perfusion of vital organs.

2. Signs and symptoms :
They can vary, but often include :
  * Fever or hypothermia
  * Rapid, weak pulse
  * Rapid breathing
  * Low blood pressure despite appropriate treatment
  * Impaired consciousness
  * Decreased diuresis
  * Cyanosis

3. Initial treatment :
  * **Volume resuscitation:** Rapid administration of intravenous fluids is crucial to increase cardiac output and organ perfusion.
  * **Antibiotic therapy:** Antibiotics should be administered as soon as possible after culture collection to combat the underlying cause of infection.
  * **Maintenance of perfusion:** In cases where blood pressure does not respond to volume resuscitation, vasopressor drugs such as norepinephrine may be required.

4. Supervision and support of bodies :
- **Haemodynamic monitoring:** Invasive monitoring, such as an arterial catheter or Swan-Ganz catheter, may be required to assess blood pressure, cardiac output and other parameters.
- **Respiratory support:** Many patients in septic shock require mechanical ventilation due to respiratory distress or airway protection.
- **Renal support: In cases of** renal failure, extrarenal purification, such as dialysis, may be required.
- **Glycaemic control:** Controlling blood sugar levels is essential, as high or unstable levels can worsen the condition.

5. Global approach :
- **Finding the source:** Identifying and treating the source of the infection is fundamental. This may require surgery, for example to drain an abscess.
- **Laboratory monitoring:** Blood lactates, complete blood counts, cultures and biochemical tests are essential for assessing severity and guiding treatment.

Managing septic shock is a challenge that requires early recognition, rapid intervention and a multidisciplinary approach. With proper management, patients' chances of survival can be greatly improved. But it is crucial to remember that every minute counts, and that coordination between nurses, doctors and other healthcare professionals is essential to ensure the best outcome for the patient.

Intervening in a case acute renal failure

Acute renal failure (ARF) is a condition in which the kidneys suddenly lose their ability to filter waste products from the blood. It can develop in a matter of hours or days and can be fatal if not treated quickly. In intensive care, the management of AKI requires special attention and expertise.

1. Understanding acute renal failure :
AKI can result from a number of factors, including reduced blood flow to the kidneys, direct kidney damage or blockage of urine flow.

2. Common causes :
- Hypovolaemia
- Septic shock
- Nephrotoxic drugs
- Glomerulonephritis
- Obstruction of the urinary tract, as with kidney stones
- Renal ischaemia

3. Recognising signs and symptoms :
- Decreased diuresis (production of urine)
- Swelling of the legs, ankles or feet
- Fatigue or confusion
- Nausea
- Chest pain or shortness of breath
- Hyperkalaemia (high levels of potassium in the blood)

4. Intensive care unit management :
- **Restore renal perfusion:** If ARF is due to hypovolaemia or shock, the administration of intravenous fluids and/or drugs to support blood pressure may be necessary.
- **Avoid nephrotoxic drugs:** Certain drugs can aggravate ARF, so it's crucial to assess all the drugs you're taking and adjust them accordingly.
- **Careful monitoring:** Regular measurement of diuresis, blood electrolytes, creatinine and urea is essential to assess renal function and guide treatment.

- **Treatment of electrolyte imbalances:** Imbalances, particularly hyperkalaemia, can be fatal and require rapid intervention.
- **Renal support:** In serious cases where the kidneys do not rapidly recover their function, temporary extrarenal purification, such as dialysis or haemofiltration, may be necessary.

5. Working with specialists :
Early nephrological consultation is often indicated to guide treatment and make decisions about more invasive interventions such as dialysis.

Acute renal failure in intensive care requires multidisciplinary management, close monitoring and rapid intervention. The emphasis must be on prevention, treatment of the underlying cause and support for renal function. With appropriate intervention and collaboration, many cases of AKI can be reversed, allowing recovery of renal function.

Chapter 7:
EQUIPMENT AND TECHNOLOGY
IN INTENSIVE CARE

Ventilation machines and monitors

In intensive care, mechanical ventilation is often vital to support patients in respiratory distress or to protect their airways. Ventilation machines and associated monitors are central to this intervention. Understanding how they work, their modes and the parameters they monitor is essential for any professional working in intensive care.

1. Introduction to mechanical ventilation :
Mechanical ventilation is a method of replacing or supporting a patient's respiratory function by using a machine to deliver a mixture of air and oxygen directly into the lungs.

2. Ventilation machines :
   - **Constant volume ventilators:** These deliver a defined volume of air with each breath, regardless of pressure variations.
   - **Constant pressure ventilators:** They deliver air at a defined pressure, and the volume can vary according to lung compliance and airway resistance.
   - **Hybrid fans:** These combine the characteristics of the two previous fans, allowing greater flexibility in treatment.

3. Common ventilation modes :
   - **Controlled volume (CV):** A predefined volume is administered for each breath.

- **Controlled pressure (PC):** The machine delivers air until a set pressure is reached.
- **Assisted/controlled breathing (A/C):** Allows both spontaneous and mechanical breathing.
- **Pressure Support (PS):** Assists each patient's spontaneous breathing by providing predefined pressure support.
- **High-frequency ventilation:** Uses very rapid, low-volume breaths to oxygenate the lungs while minimising damage.

4. Associated monitors :
Real-time monitoring of the ventilated patient is crucial to ensuring safe and effective ventilation.
- **Tidal volume measurement:** Quantity of air delivered with each breath.
- **Airway pressure:** Indicates the pressure in the lungs during ventilation.
- **Respiratory frequency:** Number of breaths per minute, whether initiated by the patient or the machine.
- **Capnography:** Measures the concentration of exhaled CO_2, essential for assessing alveolar ventilation.
- **Oxygen saturation (SpO2):** Measures the percentage of oxygen-bound haemoglobin in the blood, reflecting the efficiency of oxygenation.

5. Practical aspects and safety :
- **Alarms:** All ventilation machines are equipped with alarms to signal deviations from set parameters, disconnections or obstructions.
- **Maintenance and checks :** Regular checks and preventive maintenance are essential to keep these vital machines running smoothly.

- **Education and training:** All professionals working in intensive care must be trained in the use, monitoring and early detection of ventilator-related problems.

Mechanical ventilation is a cornerstone of intensive care management. Mastering the technology, understanding the various ventilation modes and interpreting monitor data are essential skills to ensure safe and effective treatment. Close collaboration between doctors, nurses, respiratory therapists and technicians is essential to optimise the care of ventilated patients.

The equipment
haemodynamic monitoring

Haemodynamic monitoring is essential for assessing and guiding the management of critically ill patients in intensive care units. It provides a real-time window on the patient's cardiovascular function, enabling rapid, targeted interventions in response to haemodynamic changes.

1. Introduction to haemodynamic monitoring :
Haemodynamic monitoring enables vital parameters relating to blood circulation and cardiac function to be monitored.

2. Non-invasive monitors :
- **Non-invasive blood pressure monitor (NIBP):** Regular measurement of blood pressure using an inflatable cuff.
- **Pulse oximetry (SpO2):** Assesses blood oxygen saturation using a sensor usually placed on the fingertip.

- **Electrocardiography (ECG):** Monitors the electrical activity of the heart, enabling arrhythmias and other cardiac abnormalities to be detected.

3. Invasive monitors :
   - **Arterial catheter:** Usually placed in the radial or femoral artery, it allows continuous measurement of blood pressure and facilitates blood sampling.
   - **Swan-Ganz or pulmonary artery balloon catheter:** Inserted through a central vein and advanced into the pulmonary artery, it measures pulmonary artery pressure, central venous pressure (CVP) and cardiac output.

4. Advanced monitors :
   - **Backflow cardiometry (PICCO):** Combination of arterial catheterisation and thermodilution techniques to estimate cardiac output and other parameters.
   - **Oesophageal Doppler:** Uses ultrasound to estimate cardiac output and visualise blood flow in the main heart chambers.
   - **Bioimpedance or bioreactance monitoring:** Measures variations in the electrical resistance of the thorax to estimate blood volume and cardiac output.

5. Interpretation and application :
   - **Volume control:** use of haemodynamic data to guide fluid resuscitation and the use of vasopressors or inotropes.
   - **Assessment of cardiac function:** Detection of cardiac failure and guidance for interventions to support the heart.
   - **Monitoring after cardiac surgery:** Post-operative monitoring to detect complications and adjust therapies.

6. Safety and precautions :
- **Potential complications:** It is essential to monitor catheter insertion sites to avoid infection, haemorrhage or thrombosis.
- **Alarms:** The monitors are equipped with alarms that are triggered by deviations from defined parameters, enabling rapid intervention.
- **Training:** Intensive care nurses must be trained in the use, monitoring and rapid detection of problems associated with haemodynamic monitoring devices.

Haemodynamic monitoring is a cornerstone of patient management in intensive care. It requires a thorough understanding of the parameters being monitored, technical skills in installing and maintaining the equipment, and the ability to interpret and act on the data in real time to ensure the best possible patient management.

Technological innovations and telemedicine

In the ever-changing medical landscape of critical care, technology is playing an unprecedented role in improving patient care and facilitating collaboration between healthcare professionals. The digital age has seen the birth of telemedicine, merging medical expertise and technology to extend the reach of care, especially in situations where physical proximity is difficult.

1. Introduction to technological innovations in intensive care :
Technological advances have profoundly changed the way intensive care patients are managed, providing more precise tools for diagnosis, treatment and monitoring.

2. Electronic medical records (EMR) :
- **Centralised information:** EMRs bring together all patient information in one place, improving the efficiency and safety of care.
- **Interactivity:** They provide real-time updates, alerts for healthcare professionals and in-depth analysis of patient data.

3. Remote monitoring devices :
- **Connected monitors:** These devices send vital data to a centralised location, enabling constant monitoring, even from a distance.
- **Mobile applications:** These enable healthcare professionals to monitor patients remotely, receive alerts and consult crucial information at any time.

4. Telemedicine in intensive care :
- **Virtual consultations:** experts can intervene, offering specialist advice without being physically present next to the patient.
- **Remote monitoring:** Telemedicine centres can monitor several patients in different locations, ensuring that any anomalies are quickly identified and dealt with.
- **Education and training:** Telemedicine offers ongoing training opportunities for staff, with webinars, virtual simulations and other resources.

5. Artificial intelligence (AI) and data analysis :
- **Predicting complications:** AI algorithms can analyse patient data to identify those at risk of complications.
- **Diagnostic assistance:** AI can help detect anomalies in medical images or ECG tracings, for example.
- **Optimising management:** Analysis of large quantities of data can guide treatment decisions to maximise the chances of success.

6. Challenges and ethical considerations :
- **Data security:** Centralising data raises issues of confidentiality and security.
- **Reliability:** The adoption of new technologies requires careful verification to ensure their reliability.
- **Access and inequalities:** It is essential to ensure that the benefits of telemedicine and technological innovations reach all patients, regardless of their geographical or socio-economic situation.

The integration of technological innovations into intensive care has transformed the way care is delivered. While offering enormous benefits, these technologies require ongoing training, constant evaluation and attention to ethical issues. The challenge lies in how to integrate these tools to improve care while ensuring safety, ethics and equity for all patients.

Chapter 8:
PHARMACOLOGY IN INTENSIVE CARE

Commonly used medicines in intensive care

The complexity of managing patients in intensive care requires the use of many medicines, often powerful ones, to treat, stabilise or support vital bodily functions. This range of medicines is vast, meeting a multitude of clinical needs.

1. Introduction to drugs in intensive care :
The drugs used in intensive care are essential to respond to acute situations, organ failure and to maintain or stabilise vital parameters.

2. Cardiovascular agents :
   • **Vasopressors (noradrenaline, adrenaline):** Used to increase blood pressure in cases of severe hypotension.
   • **Inotropes (dobutamine, milrinone):** Improve cardiac contractility.
   • **Antihypertensives (nitroprusside, labetalol):** Used to reduce high blood pressure.

3. Respiratory drugs :
   • **Bronchodilators (salbutamol, ipratropium):** Dilate the airways in the event of bronchospasm.
   • Corticosteroids (hydrocortisone, methylprednisolone): Reduce pulmonary inflammation.

4. Neurological agents and sedation :
   - **Sedatives (midazolam, propofol):** Used for sedation in cases of intubation or agitation.
   - **Anticonvulsants (phenytoin, levetiracetam):** To treat or prevent epileptic seizures.
   - Analgesics (morphine, fentanyl): For pain relief.

5. Renal and electrolytic agents :
   - Diuretics (furosemide, mannitol): Help eliminate excess fluid.
   - Electrolyte supplements and correctors (potassium chloride, sodium bicarbonate): Correct electrolyte imbalances.

6. Anti-infective drugs :
   - **Antibiotics (cefazolin, meropenem):** To treat a variety of bacterial infections.
   - Antifungal agents (fluconazole, anfotericin B): To treat fungal infections.
   - Antivirals (acyclovir, oseltamivir): For viral infections.

7. Gastrointestinal drugs :
   - **Antiulcer drugs (omeprazole, ranitidine):** Protect the gastric mucosa and prevent stress ulcers.
   - **Prokinetics (metoclopramide):** Facilitate gastrointestinal motility.

8. Endocrine drugs :
   - **Insulin:** To regulate blood sugar levels.
   - **Thyroid hormones:** In certain cases of thyroid dysfunction.

9. Anticoagulants and haemostats :
   - **Heparin, warfarin:** Prevent coagulation.
   - **Protamine:** Antidote to heparin.
   - **Coagulation factors:** In the event of bleeding or coagulopathy.

Managing drugs in intensive care is crucial for the nursing staff. Each agent has its own indications, contraindications, interactions and side effects. Judicious use, based on a thorough understanding, guarantees optimal management and minimises the risks associated with medication.

Administration and management side effects

Effective drug administration is an essential component of resuscitation care. However, due to the potency and complexity of the drugs used, the monitoring and management of side effects is just as crucial in ensuring patient safety and well-being.

1. Introduction :
Managing medicines in intensive care goes beyond simple administration. It involves constant monitoring of patient responses, early detection of adverse effects and rapid intervention to mitigate these effects.

2. Administration protocols :
- **Pre-administration check:** to ensure that the right drug is given to the right patient, in the right dose, by the right route, at the right time.
- **Administration techniques:** the specific knowledge needed to administer drugs by various routes, such as intravenous, oral or inhaled.
- **Post-administration monitoring:** Immediate monitoring after administration to detect any signs of reaction.

3. Common side effects :
- **Allergic reactions:** Symptoms such as skin rashes, oedema, dyspnoea or anaphylactic shock.

- **Organ-specific toxicities:** For example, nephrotoxicity with certain antibiotics or cardiotoxicity with certain drugs.
- **Effects on the central nervous system:** Drowsiness, dizziness or agitation with certain analgesics or sedatives.

4. Prevention of side effects :
- **Titration:** Adjusting the dose to obtain the desired effect without side effects.
- **Therapeutic monitoring:** Use laboratory tests to monitor drug levels, particularly those with a narrow therapeutic margin.
- **Patient education:** Informing patients (where possible) and their families of potential side-effects so that they can be detected early.

5. Response to side effects :
- **Dose adjustment:** Reduce or increase the dose depending on the situation.
- **Antidotes:** Some drugs have specific antidotes to counter their effects.
- **Symptomatic support:** For example, administering antihistamines for an allergic reaction.

6. Psychological and emotional implications :
- **Anxiety and confusion:** Some drugs can induce altered mental states. Recognition and mitigation of these effects are crucial.
- **Communication:** Explain to the family and the patient (if possible) the reasons for changes in mood or behaviour due to medication.

7. Interprofessional collaboration :
- **Role of the pharmacist:** Pharmacists are invaluable allies in helping to optimise the administration of

medicines, providing information on drug interactions and advising on the management of side effects.

- **Interdisciplinary teams:** Collaboration between nurses, doctors, pharmacists and other healthcare professionals is essential for optimal drug management.

Managing side effects in intensive care requires rigorous monitoring, rapid intervention and close collaboration between healthcare professionals. Every medicine has the potential to bring a therapeutic benefit, but it is essential to weigh up these benefits against the potential risks. The main objective is always to ensure the safety, comfort and well-being of the patient.

Antibiotic prophylaxis and infection management

One of the major challenges in intensive care is the prevention and management of infections. Antibiotic prophylaxis, the use of antibiotics to prevent infections, plays an essential role in this respect. However, the right approach requires a delicate balance between preventing infections and limiting antibiotic resistance.

1. Introduction:
The intensive care environment is particularly prone to infections: critically ill patients, frequent invasive procedures, and a high rate of antibiotic use. Hence the importance of antibiotic prophylaxis and effective infection management.

2. Principles of antibiotic prophylaxis :
- **Targeting:** Antibiotic prophylaxis is not universal; it is used for specific situations or procedures with a high risk of infection.

- **Duration:** This is generally of short duration to limit the development of resistance.
- **Choice of antibiotic:** The antibiotic must be effective against the most likely pathogens for the procedure or situation concerned.

3. Situations requiring antibiotic prophylaxis :
   - **High-risk surgery:** e.g. cardiovascular procedures, transplants.
   - **Serious trauma:** open fractures, craniocerebral trauma.
   - Insertion of invasive medical devices: central catheters, drains.

4. Recognition and monitoring of infections :
   - **Clinical signs:** Fever, leukocytosis, changes in blood pressure.
   - **Microbiological examination:** blood cultures, urine cultures, body fluid cultures.

5. Management of known infections :
   - **Rapid initiation of treatment :** Rapid administration of antibiotics is often vital.
   - **Adaptive therapy:** Adjustment of treatment based on the sensitivity of the pathogens identified.
   - **Sequential therapy:** Switching from intravenous to oral therapy as soon as the patient is stable.

6. Preventing healthcare-associated infections :
   - **Hand hygiene:** The simplest and most effective measure for preventing the transmission of infections.
   - **Isolation precautions:** In the case of patients infected or colonised by resistant pathogens.

7. The problem of multi-resistant bacteria:
   - **Surveillance:** Rapid detection of colonisation or infection by resistant strains is essential.

- **Control strategies:** isolation of patients, reinforced disinfection, and limiting the use of broad-spectrum antibiotics.

8. Education and training :
- **Medical team:** Raising awareness of good hygiene practices, antibiotic prophylaxis protocols and antibiotic management.
- **Patients and families:** Raising awareness of the importance of hand hygiene and recognising the signs of infection.

Antibiotic prophylaxis and infection management in the intensive care unit are a real challenge, requiring a multifaceted approach. The aim is twofold: to protect patients from infection while preserving the effectiveness of antibiotics for the future.

Chapter 9:
Ethics AND LEGISLATION IN INTENSIVE CARE

End-of-life decisions and limiting care

In the hectic world of intensive care, where life constantly rubs shoulders with death, end-of-life decisions and limiting care are among the most delicate and emotional challenges for the medical team, patients and their families.

1. Introduction:
Faced with situations where recovery is no longer possible or where medical interventions may prolong life without improving its quality, healthcare professionals are called upon to make complex end-of-life decisions.

2. Ethics and guiding principles :
- **Autonomy:** Respecting the patient's wishes and preferences, where these are known.
- **Benefit and non-benefit:** Weighing up the benefits and risks of treatments.
- **Justice:** Ensuring that resources are used fairly and that each patient receives appropriate care.

3. Communication :
- **Early discussion:** Discuss the patient's wishes and preferences well before the situation becomes critical.
- **Open dialogue:** Ensure transparent communication with the patient (where possible) and family about the patient's condition, treatment options and expected outcomes.

4. Limitation of care :
- **Not to undertake:** Choosing not to begin a treatment or intervention because of its presumed uselessness or the patient's wishes.
- **Discontinue:** Discontinue a treatment or procedure that is already underway because it is deemed unnecessary or contrary to the patient's wishes.

5. Palliative sedation :
- **Objective: To** relieve unbearable symptoms at the end of life, such as pain or anxiety, without the intention of hastening death.
- **Methods:** Choice of medication, adjustment of doses and monitoring of effects.

6. Refusal of treatment by the patient :
- **The patient's right:** Everyone has the right to refuse treatment, even if this may result in death.
- **Advance directives :** Document written by the patient, expressing his/her wishes concerning his/her care at the end of life.

7. Supporting the family :
- **Emotional support:** Helping the family to get through this difficult period and to mourn.
- **Inclusion in decision-making:** Involving the family in decision-making, while respecting the patient's wishes.

8. The aftermath: grief and support :
- **Debriefing:** Post-mortem discussions with the medical team to understand the decisions taken.
- **Psychological support:** offering counselling or therapy sessions to help deal with bereavement.

9. Training and support for the medical team :
- **Ethics training:** Regular training for the team on ethical principles and best practice in end-of-life decisions.
- **Emotional support:** Providing a space where team members can express their emotions and receive support.

End-of-life decisions in intensive care are profoundly human, requiring careful listening, deep compassion and a strong sense of ethics. By respecting the patient's wishes and dignity, while supporting the family and the medical team, these decisions can be taken with integrity and humanity.

Legislation on organ donation

Organ donation is one of the most delicate and complex areas of medicine. In the context of intensive care, the possibility of harvesting organs for transplantation may arise following a situation where brain death has been declared, raising a series of ethical, practical and legal questions.

1. Introduction :
Organ donation saves lives every day. However, behind each altruistic gesture lie regulatory and legislative aspects designed to guarantee the safety, respect and dignity of both donor and recipient.

2. Key definitions :
- **Cerebral death:** Total and irreversible absence of all cerebral activity.
- **Living donor: An** individual who donates an organ or part of an organ during their lifetime.

- **Deceased donor: A** person who has suffered brain death or cardiocirculatory death.

3. Consent to the donation :
   - **Presumed consent:** In some countries, every citizen is presumed to be a donor unless they have explicitly objected during their lifetime.
   - **Explicit consent:** System in which post-mortem organ donation requires prior authorisation from the donor or the donor's family.

4. The role of the family :
   - **Information:** Informing the family of the potential for organ donation, while respecting their need to grieve.
   - **Decision:** If the deceased has not expressed his or her wishes, the family is often consulted to make the decision.

5. Procedure for declaring brain death :
   - **Neurological tests:** Tests to confirm the total absence of brain activity.
   - **Documentation:** All declarations of brain death must be meticulously documented.

6. Safety and ethics of sampling :
   - **Absence of conflict of interest:** The intensive care team responsible for the patient must be separate from the transplant team.
   - **Respect for the body:** Procedures must be carried out with care to guarantee the donor's dignity.

7. Allocation of organs :
   - **Fairness:** Organs must be allocated on the basis of medical need, not socio-economic criteria.
   - **Compatibility:** Ensuring a match between donor and recipient to maximise the chances of a successful transplant.

8. Organ donation from living donors :
  - Medical and psychological assessment: To guarantee the safety of the donor.
  - **Free and informed consent:** The donor must be fully informed of the risks and benefits.

9. Awareness-raising and education :
  - **National campaigns:** to encourage people to express their wishes regarding organ donation.
  - **Medical training:** Train healthcare professionals to approach the subject with tact and compassion.

The legislation surrounding organ donation is at a crossroads between the medical imperative to save lives and the ethical imperative to respect the will and dignity of individuals. Clarity, transparency and compassion must guide every step of the process, from the declaration of brain death to successful transplantation.

Confidentiality and informed consent

Medicine, at the intersection of science, ethics and humanity, constantly reminds us that each patient is a unique entity, worthy of respect and attention. Two of the pillars of this delicate dance between healthcare professionals and patients are confidentiality and informed consent. These concepts, although familiar, become more complex as we get to the heart of the matter.

From the very first contact with a patient, a kind of tacit contract is established. This contract guarantees that everything that is shared, discussed or observed will remain within the walls of the practice or examination room. Confidentiality is this silent promise that the doctor makes to the patient: a promise of discretion, security and respect. It is a protection, not only for the intimate details of the patient's health, but also for their dignity, reputation and, sometimes, their deepest fears. In a world where information is a currency, confidentiality is a fortress.

But medicine is more than listening and observing. It requires action, intervention and decisions. And that's where informed consent comes in. Let's imagine for a moment that medicine is a vast sea, rich in possibilities but strewn with potential storms. Informed consent is the patient's compass for navigating this sea. It ensures that the patient understands not only the calm waters ahead, but also the potential storms. So when the doctor proposes a route, the patient is in a position to accept or refuse it, armed with all the necessary information.

The informed consent process is a delicate dance. The doctor must not only inform, but also ensure that the patient really understands. It is not a simple formality, but an open and continuous dialogue. It's an invitation to ask questions, express doubts and share concerns. It's a recognition that, while the doctor is the expert on medicine, the patient is the expert on his or her own life.

There are, of course, times when these principles are put to the test: emergency situations where time is of the essence, times when the patient's ability to understand is compromised, or situations where relatives have to intervene. But these exceptions only serve to underline the importance of these pillars in everyday practice.

Ultimately, confidentiality and informed consent are not just concepts or procedures. They reflect the profound humanity of medicine. They are a reminder that, at the heart of every intervention, every diagnosis, every treatment, there is a person - with his or her hopes, fears, dreams and concerns. And it is this person, in all his or her complexity and uniqueness, who must always remain at the centre of the medical equation.

Chapter 10:
RESEARCH AND ADVANCES
IN INTENSIVE CARE

Clinical studies :
understand and participate

The world of medicine is constantly evolving, drawing on scientific discoveries and advances to constantly improve patient care. At the heart of these advances are clinical trials. This medical research, carried out on volunteers, is used to develop new treatments, test their effectiveness and ensure their safety. However, involvement in a clinical trial can raise questions and even concerns. Understanding their essence and process is therefore crucial for anyone considering taking part.

First of all, it's important to define what a clinical trial is. Imagine a bridge between laboratory research, where new molecules or techniques are discovered, and the hospital room where a patient receives treatment. This bridge is the clinical trial. It validates that the treatment is not only effective, but also safe for the patient.

Clinical trials generally take place in several phases. The main aim of the first phase is to determine the safety of a treatment, identify potential side effects and establish the optimal dosage. Subsequent phases gradually expand the group of participants to assess the efficacy of the treatment, compare it with other existing treatments and monitor long-term side effects. Each phase is rigorously guided by strict protocols, guaranteeing the safety and well-being of the participants.

But why choose to take part in a clinical trial? The reasons vary. For some, it's the hope of gaining access to a new treatment that is potentially more effective than current options. For others, it's the altruistic desire to contribute to the progress of medicine. However, this decision should never be taken lightly. Participation involves commitments, such as regular medical visits, tests or treatment adjustments. What's more, like all research, results are not guaranteed. Some participants may experience significant improvements, while others may not.

This is where the importance of informed consent comes in. Before taking part in a study, each volunteer must be fully informed of the objectives, procedures, potential risks and expected benefits. This process ensures that the decision to participate is based on a full understanding and not on false expectations or misunderstandings.
It is also essential to understand that each participant has the right to withdraw from a clinical study at any time, without any negative consequences for their future medical care.

Clinical trials are invaluable tools in medicine's never-ending journey towards new horizons. They embody the collaboration between researchers, healthcare professionals and patients to write the next chapters of modern medicine. For those considering taking part, it is essential to get informed, ask questions and weigh up the pros and cons carefully, because in this quest for progress, every participant is a valuable partner.

The latest discoveries and major advances in intensive care

Intensive care is the crucible where life often oscillates between fragility and resilience. Over time, this medical speciality has benefited from major innovations and discoveries that have not only improved patient care, but have also shaped the future of emergency medicine. Let's take a look at some of the most significant advances in resuscitation in recent years.

- Personalised medicine in intensive care :
    - Advances in genomics and bioinformatics have led to a better understanding of how individual genetic factors can influence a patient's response to treatment. This has led to more targeted and individualised treatments for intensive care patients, minimising side effects and optimising outcomes.
- Telemedicine in intensive care :
    - The advent of telemedicine has enabled resuscitation experts to advise and assist medical teams remotely, particularly in underserved areas or during health crises such as the COVID-19 pandemic.
- Advances in mechanical ventilation :
    - Innovations in ventilation machines have led to more adaptive ventilation modes that respond in real time to the patient's needs, thereby reducing ventilation-related complications.
- ECMO (Extracorporeal Membrane Oxygenation) :
    - Although ECMO is not entirely new, its applications and techniques have improved, offering a lifeline to patients with severe heart or lung failure when other interventions have failed.
- Targeted temperature management :
    - Research has shown that precise control of body temperature after cardiac arrest can improve neurological outcomes. This has led to wider adoption of hypothermic therapy and targeted thermal management.

- Biomarkers in intensive care :
    - The use of biomarkers to predict or rapidly diagnose acute conditions such as sepsis has led to faster and more targeted interventions, improving survival rates.
- Simulation in intensive care :
    - Simulation-based training for resuscitation staff has become increasingly popular, enabling practical training without risk to patients.
- Artificial intelligence (AI) and advanced   analytics :
    - AI has found its place in intensive care by helping to rapidly analyse large volumes of data, enabling early detection of organ failure or other complications.

These advances, while impressive, are only the tip of the iceberg. Resuscitation, like any other medical speciality, continues to evolve through research, innovation and the relentless dedication of healthcare professionals. As technology advances and our understanding of human biology deepens, we can expect further revolutions to transform the way we care for the most vulnerable among us.

How to stay up to date
in a constantly evolving field

In today's fast-paced world, industries, technologies and knowledge are evolving at an unprecedented rate. For any professional, staying up to date is not only a career imperative, but also a necessity if you want to offer the best of yourself. Here are some steps and strategies to help you stay at the cutting edge of your field.

- Continuing education :
  - **Courses and certifications**: Sign up for online courses, workshops or specialist training. Platforms such as Coursera, Udemy or edX offer a multitude of courses in various fields.
  - **Conferences and seminars**: These offer not only knowledge, but also networking opportunities.
- Regular reading :
  - **Trade journals**: Subscribe to the magazines and newspapers relevant to your industry.
  - **Blogs and forums**: These can provide real-time insights and practical perspectives.
- Networking :
  - Engage with colleagues, mentors and other professionals in your sector. These exchanges can often give you insights into emerging trends before they become mainstream.
- Participation in professional associations:
  - Join professional organisations related to your field. They often offer resources, training and networking opportunities.
- Use of technology :
  - **Technology watch**: Use tools like Google Alerts to keep up to date with the latest news and research in your field.
  - **Podcasts and webinars**: These are a valuable source of information and are often hosted by industry experts.
- Collaborative learning :
  - Organise or take part in study groups or discussion groups to explore new subjects or deepen existing knowledge.

- Practice and immersion :
  - Actively experiment with new methods or technologies in your day-to-day work. Learning by doing is often the most impactful.
- Make time for it:
  - Define specific times in your week to devote to your professional development. This could be as simple as reading a chapter of a book every evening or taking an online course every week.
- Mentoring :
  - Find a mentor with more experience or knowledge. Conversely, reverse mentoring (where a younger or less experienced person teaches you) can be invaluable, especially with technological trends.
- Open-mindedness :
  - Be open to change and new ideas, even if they contradict your current knowledge. Adaptability is key in a rapidly changing world.

Ultimately, staying up to date in a constantly evolving field requires a personal commitment to continuous learning. It's a never-ending journey, where the destination is professional growth and fulfilment. By adopting a proactive attitude and using the resources available, you can not only keep pace, but also become a leader in your field.

CHAPTER 11:
INFECTION MANAGEMENT
AND PRECAUTIONS

Main infections in intensive care

Intensive care units (ICUs) are highly specialised environments dedicated to the care of the most seriously ill patients. Because of the severity of their condition, the frequent use of invasive devices and the close proximity of patients to one another, nosocomial infections are a major concern in the ICU. Here is a list of the most common infections encountered in ICUs:

- Ventilator-associated pneumonia (VAP) :
    - This is the most common nosocomial infection in ICUs. It occurs in mechanically ventilated patients and is often caused by bacteria such as Pseudomonas aeruginosa, Staphylococcus aureus and Gram-negative bacteria.
- Catheter-related infections :
    - **Catheter-related bacteremias**: These are caused by contamination of central venous catheters. Microorganisms commonly involved include Staphylococcus aureus, Staphylococcus epidermidis and Gram-negative bacteria.
    - **Catheter-associated urinary tract infections**: Prolonged use of urinary catheters is a risk factor, with bacteria such as Escherichia coli and Klebsiella pneumoniae common agents.

- Surgical site infections :
    - They can develop after surgery, with bacteria such as Staphylococcus aureus, Escherichia coli or Pseudomonas aeruginosa commonly implicated.
- Abdominal infections :
    - Often due to perforations or invasive procedures, they can be caused by a variety of organisms, including Escherichia coli, Klebsiella and Bacteroides.
- Invasive mycoses :
    - Although less common than bacterial infections, fungal infections, particularly by Candida spp., can occur, particularly in immunocompromised patients or those who have received broad-spectrum antibiotic therapy.
- Sepsis and septic shock :
    - These serious conditions can result from any of the above infections and require rapid and aggressive management.
- Clostridioides difficile infections :
    - Combined with the use of antibiotics, these gastrointestinal infections can cause severe diarrhoea and other complications.
- Viral infections :
    - Although less common than bacterial infections, some viral infections, such as influenza or, more recently, COVID-19, may require ICU management.

Preventing nosocomial infections in the ICU is based on a range of measures, including rigorous hand hygiene, appropriate use of antibiotics, compliance with care protocols for invasive devices, and constant monitoring of infections.

Prevention and control measures

In the intensive care unit (ICU), infection prevention is paramount, given the vulnerability of patients and the frequent use of invasive devices. Adopting strict preventive measures can significantly reduce the risk of nosocomial infections. Here is a detailed presentation of the essential measures:

- Hand hygiene :
    - This is the simplest and most effective way of preventing the transmission of infections. It must be carried out before and after each contact with the patient, after touching potentially contaminated surfaces, before and after putting on gloves, and before any aseptic procedure.
- Standard precautions :
    - These precautions apply to all patients, whatever their pathology. They include hand hygiene, wearing gloves, masks, gowns and eye protection where there is a risk of splashing, and safe management of waste and soiled linen.
- Additional precautions :
    - Depending on the type of pathogen, additional measures may be required, such as patient isolation, the installation of airlocks or the use of specific protective equipment.
- Maintenance of invasive devices :
    - The insertion, maintenance and removal of these devices must follow strict protocols to reduce the risk of infection. This applies in particular to catheters, urinary catheters and airways.

- Infection surveillance :
  - Setting up a monitoring system means that any epidemic can be identified quickly and protocols adjusted accordingly.
- Antibiotic strategy :
  - Judicious use of antibiotics is essential to prevent the emergence of resistant bacteria. This includes prescribing antibiotics only when necessary, selecting the right antibiotic and administering it for the right length of time.
- Cleaning and disinfection :
  - Surfaces, equipment and the ICU environment must be regularly cleaned and disinfected according to defined protocols.
- Training and education :
  - Staff must be regularly trained and informed about best practice in infection prevention.
- Vaccination :
  - Healthcare staff must be up to date with their vaccinations to prevent the transmission of preventable diseases.
- Communication :
  - Open communication between team members is essential to ensure that protocols are followed and that any abnormality or suspected infection is promptly reported.
- Patient and family involvement:
  - Patients and their relatives can be involved in preventive measures, by being informed of the risks, the signs of infection and the hygiene measures to adopt.

Strict implementation and compliance with these measures, combined with constant monitoring, are the key to minimising the risk of nosocomial infections in intensive care units.

Antibiotic resistance : a major challenge

In today's complex panorama of medical challenges, antibiotic resistance stands out as one of the most urgent and pervasive threats to public health. Within the sterile walls of intensive care units, this resistance is particularly acute. Let us delve into the heart of this issue.

- Genesis of resistance :
  - Antibiotic resistance is not a new phenomenon; it has existed since the very emergence of antibiotics. In fact, every time a bacterium is exposed to an antibiotic, it undergoes selective pressure. Susceptible bacteria die off, while resistant bacteria, thanks to genetic mutations, survive and multiply. With time and the inappropriate use of antibiotics, this resistance has increased.
- Consequences in intensive care :
  - Patients in intensive care are often seriously ill and vulnerable. An infection with resistant bacteria can seriously complicate their management, prolong their stay in hospital, and increase mortality and the cost of care.
- Superbugs":
  - Bacteria such as MRSA (methicillin-resistant Staphylococcus aureus), VRE (vancomycin-resistant Enterococci), and carbapenemase-producing bacteria threaten ICUs around the world. These superbugs can be resistant to several classes of antibiotics, making therapeutic options limited.
- Contributing factors :
  - The over-prescription of antibiotics, the use of broad-spectrum antibiotics when a narrow spectrum would suffice, the inadequate duration of treatment and the inappropriate use

of antibiotics in veterinary medicine and agriculture all contribute to the emergence of resistance.
- Prevention is the key:
  - Raising doctors ' awareness of responsible prescribing, using bacterial cultures to guide the choice of antibiotic, rotating antibiotics in hospitals and implementing antibiotic therapy protocols are all essential measures.
- Research and development :
  - In the face of growing resistance, it is imperative to develop new antibiotics. However, development is slow and costly, requiring a global commitment.
- International collaboration :
  - Antibiotic resistance is a global problem. International collaboration to monitor resistance and share information and best practice is essential.
- Education and awareness :
  - Patients, carers and the general public need to be informed about the importance of using antibiotics appropriately and the risks associated with their misuse.

Antibiotic resistance in intensive care represents a monumental challenge. However, with collaborative efforts, increased awareness, judicious use of antibiotics and a renewed impetus in research, we can hope to counter this threat and continue to offer quality care to the most vulnerable patients.

Chapter 12:
NUTRITION AND METABOLIC SUPPORT

The importance of nutrition
in intensive care

In resuscitation, the art of saving lives is not limited to mastering sophisticated machines or administering powerful drugs. One of the fundamental, often underestimated but crucial elements is nutrition. Much more than a simple food intake, nutrition in the intensive care unit is a delicate science that plays a decisive role in patient recovery.

- Nutrition: a vital function :
    - Nutrition ensures the necessary intake of macronutrients (proteins, carbohydrates, lipids) and micronutrients (vitamins, minerals), which are essential for maintaining bodily functions, supporting healing and preventing complications.
- Impact on recovery :
    - The right nutritional intake can improve the immune response, preserve muscle mass, reduce the catabolism (breakdown) induced by the disease and speed up recovery.
- The challenges of nutrition in intensive care :
    - Patients in intensive care may have specific nutritional needs due to their state of health, the severity of their illness or co-morbidities. In addition, pathological processes such as inflammation or sepsis can modify metabolism, making it complex to determine nutritional requirements.

- Methods of administration :
  - The enteral route (through the digestive tract) is preferred whenever possible, as it maintains the integrity of the intestinal mucosa and presents a lower risk of infection. However, in some cases, parenteral nutrition (intravenous administration) may be necessary.
- Close monitoring :
  - Patients' nutritional status must be assessed regularly, using clinical, biochemical and anthropometric parameters. This makes it possible to adjust intakes according to the patient's progress.
- Risks of malnutrition :
  - Inadequate or inappropriate nutrition can lead to muscle loss, reduced immune defences, increased infectious complications and slower recovery.
- Multidisciplinary collaboration :
  - Effective nutritional management requires collaboration between doctors, nurses, dieticians and pharmacists. Each professional contributes his or her expertise to the development of a tailored nutritional plan.
- Education and research :
  - As with all aspects of intensive care, ongoing training and research are essential to ensure optimal nutritional management, based on the latest scientific discoveries.

In the hustle and bustle of intensive care units, where every second counts, nutrition can seem a secondary consideration. Yet it is one of the cornerstones of care, a real pillar that supports patients' healing and recovery. As Hippocrates put it so well: "Let your food be your first medicine". In the context of resuscitation, these words have never been more relevant.

Route of administration and special schemes

The world of resuscitation is so complex that every decision, every action, has profound implications for the patient. Among these fundamental decisions, the way we administer nutrition and the specific diets we adopt according to the patient's unique needs play a predominant role.

- Route of administration :
    - Enteral :
    - This is the preferred   route, using the patient's own digestive system. It is less invasive, preserves the function and structure of the intestine and reduces the risk of associated infections.
    - Sub-categories: Nasogastric tube, nasoduodenal tube, nasojejunal tube, gastrostomy or jejunostomy.
    - Parenteral :
    - Used when enteral feeding is not possible or insufficient. It involves administering nutrients directly into the bloodstream.
    - Sub-categories: Central parenteral nutrition, peripheral parenteral nutrition.
- Special schemes :
    - Standard :
    - For patients who have   no specific needs or underlying illnesses affecting their nutritional requirements.
    - High calorie :
    - For patients with increased energy requirements, such as those with significant weight loss or high metabolic needs.

- Low-calorie :
- For obese   patients or those at risk of fluid overload.
- Diabetics:
- To manage and control blood sugar levels in diabetic patients or those at risk.
- Renal diet :
- Suitable for patients with kidney disease or renal insufficiency, with adjustments for protein, potassium, phosphorus and sodium.
- Hepatic :
- For patients with liver disease, this diet modifies the intake of proteins, electrolytes and fluids.
- Factors to consider :
  - The patient's energy metabolism, fluid balance, renal and hepatic function, gastrointestinal status and other parameters must be closely monitored in order to adjust the diet.
  - Food allergies, intolerances and patient preferences must also be taken into account when planning.
- Monitoring and complications :
  - Regular monitoring of intakes and tolerances is essential to prevent associated complications, whether mechanical (e.g. displacement of a catheter), metabolic or infectious.
- Multidisciplinary team :
  - Collaboration between doctors, nurses, dieticians and other health professionals is crucial to developing a suitable nutritional plan and ensuring ongoing monitoring.
- Evolution of the plan :
  - Depending on the patient's condition, the diet may need to be adapted, modified or

discontinued. Regular reassessment is therefore essential to ensure that the diet meets the patient's changing needs.

Nutrition is much more than just food, it is a precise and delicate science in intensive care. Routes of administration and specific diets must be chosen carefully, taking into account the unique condition of each patient, in order to promote optimal recovery.

Complication management linked to nutrition

Nutrition in the intensive care unit is an essential pillar of patient management, but it is not without its challenges. Like any medical intervention, nutrition, whether enteral or parenteral, can be associated with complications. Knowing how to anticipate, recognise and respond to them is vital to guaranteeing the patient's well-being.

- Complications of the enteral route :
  - Obstruction of the probe :
    - Prevention: Regularly flush the probe with water.
    - Intervention: Use enzymatic or bicarbonate solutions to dislodge obstructions.
  - Moving the probe :
    - Prevention: Fix the probe correctly and check its position regularly.
    - Intervention: Reintroduce or replace the catheter, if necessary, under radiographic or endoscopic guidance.

- Reflux and suction :
    - Prevention: Elevate the head of the bed, check the gastric residue, adapt the infusion speed.
    - Intervention: Aspirate secretions, assess the need for antibiotics and consider post-pyloric nutrition.
- Diarrhoea or constipation:
    - Prevention: Choose a suitable formula, assess tolerance and monitor medications that affect intestinal motility.
    - Intervention: Adjust the formula, consider pro- or anti-motility drugs as required.
- Complications of the parenteral route :
    - Infections :
        - Prevention: Use aseptic techniques and change catheters and tubing regularly.
        - Intervention: Cultivate the insertion site, administer antibiotics, consider removing the catheter.
    - Metabolic complications :
        - Prevention: Closely monitor electrolytes, blood sugar, kidney and liver function.
        - Intervention: Adjust the composition of the parenteral solution, administer corrective medication.
    - Thrombosis or embolism :
        - Prevention: Assess the risk, consider prophylactic anticoagulation.
        - Intervention: administer anticoagulants, consider removing the catheter, and in serious cases, consider surgery.
- Allergic reactions :
    - Prevention: Know the patient's allergies, check the composition of formulas.

- Intervention: Stop administration, treat allergic reaction with antihistamines, steroids or adrenaline depending on severity.
- Intolerance to the formula :
  - Prevention: Start with low volumes and increase gradually, monitor tolerance.
  - Intervention: Adjust the formula or infusion speed, consider medication to treat symptoms.

Managing nutrition-related complications requires careful monitoring, rapid intervention and close collaboration between members of the healthcare team. By being vigilant, educating patients and their families, and working together, we can maximise the benefits of nutrition while minimising its risks.

Chapter 13:
INTERDISCIPLINARITY AND
ROLE OF OTHER PROFESSIONALS

Working with physiotherapists
in intensive care

In intensive care, a multidisciplinary approach is at the heart of patient care. Physiotherapists are one of the key players in this team, playing a vital role in patient recovery and well-being. Their expertise helps not only to improve physical function, but also to prevent potentially fatal complications.

- The role of the physiotherapist in intensive care :
  - Respiratory rehabilitation :
    - Bronchial drainage techniques to help clear secretions.
    - Breathing techniques to improve gas exchange and oxygenation.
    - Teaching productive coughing to avoid the accumulation of secretions.
  - Early mobilisation :
    - Avoid muscle atrophy and the complications of prolonged immobilisation.
    - Passive, semi-active and active mobilisation techniques depending on the patient's abilities.
  - Positioning :
    - Prevention of pressure sores and contractures.
    - Optimising respiratory function through regular changes of position.

- Working with the care team :
  - Daily planning :
    - Define objectives for each patient with doctors, nurses and other professionals.
    - Adapt interventions according to the patient's clinical condition.
  - Training and education :
    - Raising the team 's awareness of the importance of early mobilisation and breathing techniques.
    - Educate patients and their families about techniques they can practise themselves.
- Specific challenges and considerations :
  - Hemodynamic stability :
    - Adapting interventions according to the patient's vital parameters and stability.
    - Working closely with nurses to monitor vital signs during sessions.
  - Sedation and analgesia :
    - Communicate with doctors to adjust sedation so that the patient can participate actively.
    - Strike a balance between reducing pain and enabling the patient to participate actively in the sessions.
  - Medical equipment :
    - Manoeuvre carefully around pipes, drains and catheters to avoid accidental disconnection.
- Impact on recovery :
  - Physiotherapy in intensive care has been shown to speed up recovery, reduce the length of stay in intensive care and in hospital, and improve quality of life after discharge.

The intensive care physiotherapist is an essential link in the care chain. Their ability to work hand in hand with other healthcare professionals, while focusing on the unique needs of each patient, contributes significantly to improving the outcomes and well-being of critically ill patients.

The role of psychologists and psychiatrists in intensive care units

In the complex and often stressful environment of the intensive care unit (ICU), psychological support is of crucial importance. Patients, their families and even staff can be confronted with emotionally charged situations. This is where psychologists and psychiatrists come in, providing invaluable expertise in navigating the tumultuous waters of emotions and the mind.

- For patients:
    - Trauma of hospitalisation :
        - Some patients may experience the ICU as a shock, with feelings of uncertainty, fear and helplessness. Psychologists can help them deal with these emotions.
    - Delusions and confusion :
        - Confusion syndrome in the ICU is common and can be very disruptive. Psychiatrists can play a part in its management, both with and without medication.
    - Preparing for the sequel :
        - Helping patients to understand the next steps in their recovery and to manage any anxiety or depression that may ensue.

89

- For families :
  - Stress and bereavement management :
    - Faced with the serious illness of a loved one, families may feel shock, anger, sadness or helplessness. Psychological support can help them through these difficult times.
  - Communication :
    - Psychologists can facilitate communication between Caregiver staff and families, helping to clarify information and manage expectations.
- For staff :
  - Burn-out :
    - ICU staff are often faced with life-and-death situations, which can lead to intense stress. Psychologists and psychiatrists can offer interventions and strategies to manage stress and prevent burn-out.
  - Debriefings after critical incidents:
    - After traumatic events or losses in the ICU, debriefing sessions can be organised to help the team process emotions and reactions.
  - Training :
    - Psychologists can offer training in communication, stress management and other psychosocial skills.
  - Research and development :
    - Psychiatrists and psychologists may also be involved in ICU research, investigating the best methods of supporting patients, families and staff.

The presence of mental health professionals in the ICU is not simply a luxury, but a necessity. They play a pivotal role in overall care, ensuring that the mental and emotional aspect is addressed with as much care and expertise as the physical aspect. Ultimately, it is this holistic approach that guarantees the best results for patients and a better quality of work for staff.

Working with social workers and the ethics team

The intensive care unit (ICU) is an environment where medical, social and ethical dilemmas are commonplace. In this dynamic, social workers and the ethics team play a fundamental role in ensuring comprehensive and balanced patient care. Their work in tandem with the medical team is essential in meeting the complex needs of patients and their families.

- Role   of social workers :
    - Psychosocial assessment :
        - The social workers carry   o u t   a comprehensive assessment of the needs and concerns of patients and their families, ranging from financial issues to access to care after the ICU stay.
    - Emotional   support :
        - They offer emotional   s u p p o r t, helping families navigate the maze of emotions and decisions associated with a stay in the ICU.
    - Coordination of resources :
        - Whether organising transport, rehabilitation or care at home, social workers are the bridge between the hospital and community services.

- Mediation :
  - In the event of conflict or misunderstanding between medical staff and the family, they can act as mediators to facilitate communication.
- Role of the ethics team :
  - Ethical dilemmas :
    - The team intervenes when ethical issues arise, such as end-of-life decisions, informed consent or limiting care.
  - Consultations :
    - The team offers consultations to healthcare professionals and families to discuss and clarify ethical dilemmas.
  - Training :
    - It provides training for ICU staff on current ethical issues and best practice in dealing with them.
  - Recommendations:
    - Based on ethical principles, the team can make recommendations on the best course of action in complex situations.
- Collaboration between social workers, ethics team and medical staff:
  - Interdisciplinary meetings :
    - Regular meetings allow us to discuss specific cases, share perspectives and make balanced decisions.
  - Care planning :
    - By combining medical, ethical and social skills, the team can develop a care plan that takes into account all aspects of the patient's well-being.
  - Raising awareness and continuing education :
    - Joint sessions can be organised to raise awareness and train all staff on ethical and social issues in the ICU.

Collaboration between social workers, the ethics team and the rest of the medical staff enhances the quality of care in the ICU. By ensuring that each patient is seen not only as a set of medical symptoms, but also as a person with needs, concerns and rights, this collaboration guarantees a holistic approach that respects the dignity of each individual.

Chapter 14:
CONTINUING EDUCATION
AND THE OUTLOOK FOR THE FUTURE

The need for an update
regular skills development

In the fast-paced and ever-changing world of medicine, the need to regularly update skills has never been more crucial, particularly in demanding areas such as the intensive care unit (ICU). As technological advances and scientific discoveries transform medical practice, healthcare professionals are faced with the constant challenge of staying at the cutting edge of their speciality.

- The dynamic nature of medicine :
  - Clinical discoveries, new treatment methods, innovative medicines and technological advances regularly revolutionise medical practice. Without ongoing training, healthcare professionals run the risk of being overwhelmed by out-of-date information, thereby compromising the quality of care offered to patients.
- The importance of precision in the ICU :
  - In an environment where every decision can have vital consequences, it is imperative to be informed about current best practice. A simple error or lack of information can have devastating consequences.
- Meeting the expectations of patients and families:
  - In an age of information, patients and their families are increasingly well-informed and have high expectations of care. A professional

with up-to-date knowledge and skills inspires confidence and credibility.
- Professional regulations and standards :
  - Regulatory bodies and professional associations often set standards that require ongoing training. Failure to comply with these requirements may have legal and professional implications.
- Professional development and satisfaction :
  - In addition to the benefits for patients, regular updating of skills enhances the sense of achievement and job satisfaction. It also opens doors to career, research and leadership opportunities.
- Interdisciplinary collaboration :
  - As roles within medical teams evolve, understanding the latest skills and knowledge in each specialty facilitates collaboration and improves patient-centred care.

How to ensure regular updates :
- **Training and workshops**: Regular participation in training courses, conferences and workshops specific to the speciality.
- **Reading**: Follow renowned medical journals, magazines and other relevant publications.
- **Professional networks**: Exchanging with colleagues, joining professional associations and taking part in specialist discussion forums.
- **Certifications**: Regular certification or recertification in specialist areas.
- **Feedback**: Actively seek feedback from colleagues, mentors and even patients.

Ultimately, updating skills is at the heart of patient-centred medicine. Not only does it guarantee optimal care, it also reinforces the confidence, integrity and professionalism of the carer. In the demanding world of the ICU, this is an absolute requirement for every professional aspiring to excellence.

Specialisations in intensive care

Intensive care, the medical field par excellence for the care of critically ill patients, requires a high level of expertise. While the general intensive care unit (ICU) deals with a wide range of pathologies, numerous specialisations have emerged to meet the specific needs of certain groups of patients. These specialities offer more advanced training and expertise, enabling patients to be cared for in the best possible way.

- Cardiovascular resuscitation :
  - **Special features**: Focus on patients with severe cardiac conditions, from acute heart failure to complex arrhythmias.
  - **Common interventions**: Cardiac catheterisation, haemodynamic support such as counter-pulsation balloons or ECMO.

- Neurological resuscitation :
  - **Special features**: Care for patients with critical neurological conditions such as stroke, head trauma or nervous system infections.
  - **Common interventions**: Monitoring intracranial pressure, therapeutic hypothermia, etc.
- Pulmonary and respiratory resuscitation :
  - **Special features**: Focus on patients with severe respiratory problems, such as ARDS (acute respiratory distress syndrome) or exacerbated COPD.

- **Common interventions**: Mechanical ventilation, bronchoscopy, veno-venous ECMO.
- Nephrology resuscitation :
  - **Special features**: Focus on patients with acute renal failure or complex electrolyte imbalances.
  - **Common interventions**: Haemodialysis, peritoneal dialysis, management of acid-base balance.
- Trauma resuscitation :
  - **Specialities**: Caring for patients who have suffered serious trauma, whether accidental or surgical.
  - **Common interventions**: Emergency airway management, emergency surgery, haemodynamic stabilisation.
- Paediatric resuscitation :
  - **Specialities**: This specialisation focuses on the care of children with serious conditions, from birth to adolescence.
  - **Common interventions**: Paediatric-specific ventilation, age-specific pharmacology, paediatric nutritional support.
- Obstetric resuscitation :
  - **Special features**: Care for pregnant women or women who have just given birth and are suffering from complications.
  - **Common interventions**: Management of post-partum haemorrhage, severe pre-eclampsia, caesarean section complications.
- Resuscitation of burn victims:
  - **Specialities**: Treatment and follow-up of patients with extensive or deep burns.
  - **Common interventions**: Airway management, reconstructive surgery, specialist wound care.

These specialisations allow a more targeted and expert approach to certain pathologies or patient populations. Nevertheless, it is essential for each specialist to remain in step with the general knowledge of intensive care, because the ICU is by its very nature a place where pathologies constantly intersect and interact.

The future of resuscitation : innovations and challenges

Intensive care, the backbone of the medical world when faced with the most critical situations, is constantly evolving. Technological advances, combined with a better understanding of diseases and pathophysiological processes, hold great promise for the years to come. But the future of intensive care also involves major challenges and ethical issues that need to be anticipated.

Firstly, **technological innovations** are at the forefront of these changes. With the emergence of artificial intelligence, numerous medical decision-making tools are being developed. They promise to guide healthcare staff towards faster, more accurate diagnoses, and to personalise treatments. Patient monitoring devices are now capable of predicting certain disorders even before they occur. Telemedicine, meanwhile, could enable better collaboration between care centres, networking expertise and guaranteeing patients access to the best skills, wherever they are.

However, as we embrace these new technologies, the importance of maintaining a patient-centred approach remains paramount. Innovation must not overshadow the human element of resuscitation. Technology is a tool, but it is healthcare professionals who provide empathy, compassion and clinical expertise.

Secondly, **ethical issues are becoming increasingly** important. With the increasing capacity to keep patients in extremely precarious states alive, when and how should decisions be made about limiting care? Euthanasia, palliative care, informed consent and taking account of patients' wishes and values are all ethical issues that arise acutely in the world of intensive care.

Furthermore, with the increase in chronic diseases and pathologies linked to an ageing population, intensive care will have to cope with growing demand. This **demographic pressure** means that we need to think about the organisation of care, staff training and the allocation of resources.

Finally, recent pandemics, such as COVID-19, have highlighted the crucial importance of intensive care units and trained professionals. Preparing for major health crises, implementing reactive protocols and conducting ongoing epidemiological research are now key concerns.

The future of intensive care is full of promise, but also full of challenges. To meet these challenges, we need to harmoniously combine the best of technology, in-depth ethical reflection and the preservation of humanity.

Chapter 15:
CONCLUSION
THE VOCATION OF THE NURSE
IN INTENSIVE CARE

The joys and challenges of the job

The job of an intensive care nurse is complex, exciting and often emotionally charged. Between moments of great satisfaction and complex situations, it's a role that demands inner strength, technical expertise and deep compassion.

The Joys :
- **Triumph over illness**: There's nothing quite like the feeling of seeing a patient, once in a critical condition, gradually recover thanks to the concerted efforts of the entire medical team. These moments remind us why so many choose this profession despite its difficulties.
- **The Patient-Caregiver Relationship** : Time spent at the bedside of an intensive care patient, particularly at times of great vulnerability, often creates strong bonds. The positive impact that a carer can have on a patient's emotional well-being is invaluable.
- **Continuous learning**: The constantly evolving nature of medicine means that every day brings new knowledge. It's a field of perpetual learning.
- **Team spirit**: Working in intensive care means working closely with a multidisciplinary team. Triumphs are shared, and challenges are overcome together.

The Challenges :
- **Loss of patients**: Despite our best efforts, some patients just don't make it. Dealing with this, and with

the bereavement of families, is one of the most difficult aspects of the job.

- **Stress and fatigue**: The days are long, sometimes unpredictable, and the workload is often intense. This can lead to physical and emotional fatigue.
- **Ethical dilemmas**: Decisions about the end of life and the withdrawal or continuation of treatment are fraught with consequences and can be a source of moral and ethical dilemmas.
- **Managing emotions**: Whether dealing with families in distress, major emergencies or complex decisions, it is essential to know how to manage your emotions while remaining effective and compassionate.
- **Rapid Technological Evolution**: Technological advances are constant in resuscitation. Keeping up to date requires an ongoing commitment to training.

Being an intensive care nurse is a whirlwind of emotions, responsibilities and learning. The challenges are great, but so are the joys and rewards. Each day brings its own share of discoveries and rewards, but also its own trials and tribulations. What remains constant is the unwavering dedication of our carers to offering their patients the very best.

Pride of service

Critical care nursing is much more than just a job. It represents a vocation, a deep passion for caring for others, even at their most vulnerable moments. Pride in the service you provide is evident in many ways, from the great victories you achieve to the more discreet gestures you make on a daily basis.

- **Restoring hope**: Patients in intensive care are often in a critical condition, sometimes on the borderline between life and death. When these patients recover, they take with them not only a second chance at life, but also deep gratitude for those who cared for them. For a nurse, knowing that he or she has played a decisive role in someone's recovery is an immense source of pride.

- **A pivotal role**: Intensive care nurses are often the first point of contact for patients and their families. Their role is not just limited to medical care, but also encompasses emotional support. Knowing that they are a pillar for their patients at such a crucial time is a responsibility that generates deep satisfaction.

- **Mastery of a unique expertise**: Intensive care requires specific knowledge and expertise. Mastering this speciality, with all its subtleties, advanced techniques and ethical challenges, is a source of great professional pride.

- **Unexpected moments of recognition**: Whether it's a thank-you from a patient, a tear from a relieved relative, or a gesture of gratitude from a colleague, these moments reinforce the profound meaning of the mission of intensive care workers.

- **Participating in a chain of life**: Every intervention, every decision taken, every smile or word of encouragement is part of a continuous chain of care aimed at saving and improving lives. This awareness of being an essential link in the chain is an undeniable source of pride.

But this pride is not without humility. It is tinged with an acute awareness of the precariousness of life, of the ephemeral nature of victories in the face of disease, and of the privileged role, but also heavy responsibility, of the intensive care nurse. It's a pride that is nurtured by the small victories of everyday life as much as the great successes, and forged in the heat of action, at the heart of the most arduous challenges of modern medicine.

Encouraging the new generation:
advice for novices

Intensive care is a world apart, requiring not only solid clinical expertise, but also great humanity. For those embarking on a career in intensive care, it's a journey full of discoveries, but also of challenges. Here's some advice for novices, to help them find their way and thrive in this demanding environment.

- **A thirst for learning**: Medicine is constantly evolving. Be insatiably curious, attend training courses and workshops, and read up on the latest research. Knowledge is one of your best allies.
- **Don't be afraid to ask questions**: Nobody has all the answers, especially at the beginning. Surround yourself with experienced colleagues and don't hesitate to ask for their help or advice.
- **Taking care of yourself**: Resuscitation can be emotionally draining. Learn to recognise the signs of fatigue, both physical and emotional, and adopt routines to recharge your batteries.
- **Cultivate empathy**: Beyond technical skills, it's your humanity that will often make the difference. Take the time to connect with your patients and their families, to understand their fears and hopes.
- **Learn from your mistakes**: You'll make mistakes, just like everyone else. The important thing is to recognise them, learn from them and constantly improve.
- **Becoming part of the team**: Resuscitation is a team effort. Get to know your colleagues, their strengths and weaknesses, and build solid relationships based on trust.
- **Give yourself time**: Mastering all the subtleties of resuscitation doesn't happen overnight. Be patient

with yourself, and remember that every day brings new skills.

- **Find mentors**: Identify experienced people who can guide, support and advise you along the way.
- **Get involved in the professional community**: Join professional associations, attend conferences and symposia. It's an excellent way of expanding your network and keeping up to date.
- **Remember why**: When the going gets tough, remember why you got into this profession in the first place. Passion, the desire to help, the satisfaction of seeing a patient recover. These reminders are essential to keep the flame burning.

For novices, it is essential to understand that resuscitation is a long-term adventure, punctuated by ups and downs, victories and challenges. Every experience, whether positive or negative, is a step towards mastering the delicate art of resuscitation care. So courage, determination and passion will be your best companions along the way.

Glossary of medical terms

The field of intensive care is full of specific medical terms. Here is a brief glossary of medical terms frequently used in intensive care. Of course, for a book, this glossary would be much more in-depth, but here is a good starting point:

- **Ablation**: surgical removal of a body part or organ.
- **Anoxia**: Total absence of oxygen in the tissues.
- **Antibiotic prophylaxis**: use of antibiotics to prevent infection.
- **Bronchoscopy**: visual examination of the airways using a bronchoscope.
- **Catheter**: flexible tube inserted into a vessel or body cavity to administer or evacuate fluids.
- **Decubitus**: Ulcer that forms when the skin and underlying tissues are compressed between a bone and a hard surface, such as a bed.
- **Electrocardiogram (ECG):** Recording of the heart's electrical activity.
- **Haemodynamics**: Study of the forces involved in blood circulation.
- **Hypoxaemia**: Decrease in the concentration of oxygen in the blood.
- **Intubation**: Insertion of a tube into the trachea to allow ventilation.
- **Bronchoalveolar lavage (BAL)**: a procedure in which a saline solution is injected into the lungs and then recovered for analysis.
- **Compensation mechanism**: Reaction of the body to restore homeostasis or balance.
- **Neurological**: Relating to the nervous system.
- **Oxygenation: The** process of bringing oxygen to the body's tissues and cells.
- **Pneumothorax**: Presence of air between the pleura and the lungs, which can lead to lung collapse.

- **Resuscitation**: the process of restoring life or consciousness, generally after cardiac arrest or respiratory failure.
- **Sedation**: Use of medication to calm a patient or make them drowsy without causing a total loss of consciousness.
- **Telemedicine:** Remote medical practice using information technology.
- **Mechanical ventilation**: Use of a ventilator to help a patient breathe.
- **Routes of administration**: Methods by which medicines are introduced into the body (oral, intravenous, intramuscular, etc.).

A detailed glossary would be essential for any student or professional seeking to deepen their knowledge in the field of resuscitation. It would provide not only definitions, but also contexts and examples to clarify the use of each term in everyday clinical practice.

Further reading and resources

Resuscitation is a complex and constantly evolving field. To stay informed and expand your knowledge, it's essential to consult relevant resources on a regular basis. Here are a few suggested readings and resources for those who want to find out more:

- Books :
    - *Principles of Critical Care* by Jesse B. Hall, Gregory A. Schmidt, and Lawrence D. H. Wood
    - *Textbook of Critical Care* by Jean-Louis Vincent, Edward Abraham, Frederick A. Moore, Patrick Kochanek, and Mitchell P. Fink
    - *The ICU Book* by Paul L. Marino
- Specialist   magazines :
    - Critical Care Medicine
    - Intensive Care Medicine
    - American Journal of Respiratory and Critical Care Medicine
    - Journal of Critical Care
- Organisations and associations :
    - *Société do Réanimation de l angue Française (SRLF)*: Provides guidelines, training and congresses on resuscitation.
    - *European Society of Intensive Care Medicine (ESICM)*: A European organisation providing resources, training and conferences on intensive care.
    - *American Thoracic Society (ATS)*: Focuses on pulmonary diseases, critical medicine and sleep.
- Online resources :
    - *Life in the Fast Lane (LITFL)*: A blog with resources on emergency medicine and resuscitation.

- *Critical Care Reviews*: Provides reviews of recent literature in critical care.
- Courses and training :
  - *Advanced Cardiovascular Life Support (ACLS)*: certification in cardiopulmonary resuscitation.
  - *Fundamental Critical Care Support (FCCS)*: Training for non-specialist intensive care professionals.
  - *European Diploma in Intensive Care (EDIC)*: European certification for doctors specialising in intensive care.
- Conferences and symposia :
  - SRLF Annual Conference
  - International Symposium on Intensive Care and Emergency Medicine (ISICEM)
- Podcasts and media :
  - *Critical Care Practitioner*: A podcast that explores various topics related to intensive care.
  - *The Bottom Line (TBL)*: A podcast that reviews and summarises critical care research articles.
- Mobile applications :
  - *MedCalX*: A medical calculator for various formulas used in intensive care.
  - *ICU Trials by ClinCalc*: An application that summarises important clinical trials in the field of intensive care.

In conclusion, resuscitation medicine is a vast and multidimensional field. Continued education and updating of knowledge is paramount to providing optimal patient care. These resources are an excellent basis on which to begin and continue this educational journey.

Books :
* Resuscitation: The reference treatise on intensive care medicine by Jean-Louis Vincent.
* *Intensive care medicine* by Jean-Daniel Chiche, Laurent Papazian and Jean-François Timsit.
* Emergency and resuscitation by Vincent Bounes.

Specialist magazines :
* *Réanimation*: Official journal of the Société de Réanimation de Langue Française (SRLF).
* *Médecine Intensive Réanimation*: Journal covering all aspects of intensive care and resuscitation.

Organisations and associations :
* *Société de Réanimation de Langue Française (SRLF):* This organisation provides recommendations and training, and organises conferences on resuscitation.
* Collège Français d'Anesthésie et de Réanimation (CFAR).

Online resources :
* *RéaNet*: A resource portal for healthcare professionals working in intensive care.
* *Urgences-Online:* Emergency information and training website.

Courses and training :
* Training in Intensive Care by the SRLF.
* Congresses on emergency medicine and resuscitation: Organised by various French-speaking bodies.

Podcasts and media :
* *RéaPod*: Podcasts focusing on intensive care medicine.
* *Flash Urgences*: A podcast focusing on emergency and intensive care.

Mobile applications :
* *SRLF*: The official application of the Société de Réanimation de Langue Française. Contains recommendations and tools for professionals.
* *RéaGuide*: Application providing technical sheets and recommendations for resuscitation practices.

Conferences and symposia :
- SRLF annual conference.
- Journées Franco-Suisses de Réanimation.

Other resources :
- *SFAR (Société Française d'Anesthésie et de Réanimation)*: This organisation also offers numerous resources, training courses and guidelines relating to resuscitation.

These resources and readings are essential for those who practise in a French-speaking environment and wish to maintain or improve their resuscitation skills.

Links to professional associations and specialised training

I'm sorry, but I can't provide direct links to websites or other online resources directly from this text. However, I can provide guidance on how to find these resources.

Professional associations :
- *French Language Resuscitation Society (SRLF)* : You can search for this organisation on Google or your preferred search engine. They have an official website which provides a wealth of information, clinical guidelines and training opportunities.
- *Collège Français d'Anesthésie et de Réanimation (CFAR)*: The official CFAR website is also a valuable source of information for professionals.
- *SFAR (Société Française d'Anesthésie et de Réanimation)*: Like other associations, they have a website where you can find guidelines, news and training opportunities.

Specialised training :
- For training, start by visiting the *SRLF* w e b s i t e . They generally offer continuing education courses and specialist workshops for resuscitation professionals.
- Universities and training institutes also offer *University Diplomas (DU)* or *Inter-University Diplomas (DIU)* in intensive care or intensive medicine. This is the case at many French medical universities.
- The *training days* and *conferences* organised by the professional associations mentioned above are also excellent opportunities for training and networking.

How do you find these resources?
- Use a search engine and enter the name of the association or training course you are interested in.
- Visit the associations' official websites for information on membership, forthcoming events and other resources.

- Consult universities or medical institutes for information on specialist resuscitation training.
- Professional social networks such as LinkedIn can also be useful for finding groups or communities dedicated to resuscitation in French.

Don't forget that the field of medicine and resuscitation is evolving rapidly, so it's crucial to keep up to date with the latest advances and training available.

www.ingramcontent.com/pod-product-compliance
Lightning Source LLC
Chambersburg PA
CBHW062332290526
45794CB00005B/2000